ESSENCE OF DAY

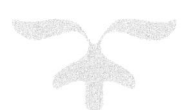

Roslyn Alexander

For the Children of Creation

Like a garden, the pages of the Bible are seeded with all kinds of plants that were quite familiar to its original audience. Roslyn Alexander invites you to join her as she strolls through Scripture, pointing out the unique properties and aromas of various plants and the spiritual insights they offer

- Susan Booth Ph-D.

Roslyn Alexander succeeded in demonstrating how exciting the Holy Scripture is and how we worship a "down to earth" God who cares about His creation. She aptly shows the theological significance of plants in the Bible to biblical teachings

- Jimmy Cobb Ph-D.

In addition to words such as "aromatic" and "Aromatherapy" already in your lexicon, get ready to add another. Let's call it, "aromatic exegesis."

Roslyn Alexander has researched and written this unique approach to understanding the Bible by focusing upon aromatic herbs, spices, and plants of the ancient Biblical world that are mentioned in the Scriptures. The book is ecologically sensitive, highly informative with regard to the botany involved, and awareness-raising to the need to have our olfactory senses engaged when we read a surprisingly large number of Biblical texts.

Contemporary Protestants and evangelicals in particular seem not to associate worship with distinct smells. This book reminds us: the ancient Hebrews certainly did! So far as I am aware, there is not another similar book in print that does what this one does with her "aromatic exegesis" approach. I do not doubt that readers will find this "olfactory hermeneutic" to be creative and downright fascinating

- Michael Fuhrman Ph-D

I love the overall approach you are taking with this writing project. I think it has great potential to reach many people. Thanks for letting me interact with the text. It is a fascinating read

- Michael Hampton Th-D.

Probably one of the best illustrations Roslyn gave (at least for me) was of her personal childhood memory for the smell of pine from her family's Christmas tree. When she gave that example, all of the sudden a number of similar examples of past memories and their aromas came to my mind. It is absolutely true that when I encounter one of those smells today, memories of both very positive and sometimes negative come back to my mind

- Salt Jones MDiv, MRE.

Roslyn Alexander has admirably presented a fascinating thread that runs through the Bible but is seldom explored: God's immense, spectacular, diverse creation of plant life and humankind's often clever, commendable management of God's gifts for a wide range of situations

- Lawson Lau Ph-D.

Written by Roslyn Alexander © 2020. All rights reserved. No part of this book may be reproduced, modified, or used in any form, including electronic, photocopying, recording, mechanical or by any information storage and retrieval system, without permission in writing from the author, except as provided by USA copyright laws.

ISBN: 9798655392397

Author Roslyn G Alexander © 2020. First submitted August 8, 2020.

Theological reviews made by:
Michael Fuhrman Ph-D.

English edit and contributions by:
James R. Lucas Ph-D.

Illustrations by Roz Gatts

Scripture references marked ESV® are taken from (The Holy Bible, English Standard Version®), copyright © 2001 by Crossway, a publishing ministry of Good News Publishers. Used by permission. All rights reserved.

Scripture references marked NIV® are taken from (The Holy Bible, New International Version®, copyright © 1973,1978, 1984, 2011, by Biblica, Inc.™ Used by permission. All rights reserved worldwide.

Holman Christian Standard Bible ® Copyright © 1999, 2000, 2003, 2009, by Holman Bible Publishers, Used with permission by Holman Bible Publishers, Nashville, Tennessee. All rights reserved.

www.facebook.com/essenceofday

Author's Introduction

Essence of Day is a study of ancient aromatic anointing oils, incense, plants and the Anointed One. This study explores how providing a fragrant offering was an important part of the Israelite or Hebraic covenant worship. Aromas with plants and burnt offerings were made in agreement with the seven most important holy days or festivals in Israel:

1) the Day of Rest (Shabbat);
2) the Festival of Unleavened Bread (Passover);
3) the day Moses presented the Torah (Shavuot) celebrated along with
4) the Festival of the Harvest (Feast of Weeks), that ends at Pentecost;
5) the Festival of Trumpets for the sounding of the New Year;
6) the Day of Atonement (Yom Kippur); and the Festival of the Booths (Sukkot) celebrated along with
7) the Festival of the First Fruits (first born). This also included animal sacrifice.

Fragrant plant compounds were used in the holy anointing oil and the holy incense which were required for covenant worship and were used in conjunction with:

* the Ark of the Covenant;
* the Lampstand;
* the Altar of Incense;
* the Table of the Bread of Presence;
* the Basin; and
* the Altar of Burnt Offering.

This has been a thought-provoking study for me. It should have a positive impact on your understanding of the tabernacle (God's dwelling place) as well as the everlasting covenant law *"as a copy and a shadow of heavenly things" (Hebrews 8:5 KJV).*

With a few exceptions, each chapter is titled after the name of a specific plant. In each chapter, the plant's properties are explored to show you how they address the human condition.

When fragrance is included along with a Scripture story, you will find that it engages the senses, reinforces listening, increases receptivity, solidifies memory impression, and provides balm for your soul.

Overview:

Today, the study of aromatic plant compounds is called "aromatherapy," or aroma science. It is primarily carried out with essential oils, specifically when they are blended for a variety of reasons. The study of aromatherapy, defined by Annette Davis, president of the National Association for Holistic Aromatherapy (NAHA), states:

> *"Aromatherapy is a part of a larger field called phytotherapy (plant therapy). True aromatherapy is the skilled use of genuine essential oils for therapeutic purposes. Science, education and experience allow aromatherapy to truly become a holistic art."*

Other experts quoted on NAHA.com include Robert Tisserand and Gabriel Mojay. According to Tisserand, Aromatherapy is beneficial *"to restore balance to the mind, body and soul."* Mojay states that Aromatherapy's purpose is *"to maintain and promote physical, psychological and spiritual well being."* (partial quotes).

This is an in-depth study of the ancient aromatic anointing oil, incense, and plants which were used for Hebraic covenant worship when aromatics had a defined role in the worship of Yahweh (which means "I-Am)". I believe aromatics and the part of our brain that interprets smells (olfaction) were designed by our Creator so that men and women might connect to a basic human need – one that we cannot fully explain when we sense, seek out, and desire a relationship with our Creator God.

Words of Knowledge and Caution:

Herbal medicine practiced in continental Europe requires a study of plant chemicals, anatomy and physiology. When taken internally, a physician must be retained to determine any potential organ toxicity and drug interactions. Please note: <u>This study does not cover the specifics and the math required for blending essential oils (referred to as EO) for either medicinal purposes or for fragrance</u>.

Each plant studied includes a section titled *historical application*, which describes some of the traditional or medicinal uses of these plants. I'm sure you'll find this most interesting. We see that all plants contain chemicals which not only make them fragrant, flavorful and useful, but which can also potentially cause an allergic reaction to our respiratory and/or integumentary system.

This study will primarily explore using fresh herbs for their fragrance. When creating a fragrance, you are practicing perfumery and learning to develop your olfactory senses, along with a vocabulary which describe specific aromas. Other professionals who use some these same skills are those who sample olive oil, honey, ale, and wine.

The author cannot be responsible for any decision you make concerning any use of essential oils. You should never replace a medical doctor's overall handling of your health care. You should definitely ask your pharmacist or doctor about possible drug interactions. Definitely consult a professional if you have any kind of allergy.

In other words, this information is not intended for your own medical adventures. "Historical use" means there has been little or no modern-day medical study or documentation regarding the effectiveness, dosage, application, or safety if you are self-diagnosing and self-treating.

The Author's Passion about this Book

With my background in occupational therapy, the fine arts, and years of studying the Scriptures, I realized that utilizing the olfactory senses, in combination with people's interest in fragrance, could enhance our learning of many Bible stories.

After studying the plants in the various Scripture passages, I noticed patterns where certain plants cropped up again and again throughout the Old and New Testaments. After I organized these short, sequential stories and combined them with a fragrance, I noticed a natural increase of interest from others as their olfactory senses became a pathway for enhanced learning.

The idea for this Bible study began in 2016 and was written in my quiet time over the past four years. But in the last year, the Lord gave it a new direction as He shed light on His word and it took root. The final edits began early in 2020 as the coronavirus pandemic began to mount.

Lord willing I intend to complete writing up lesson plans for an *Essence of Day Bible Study Workbook,* for use alongside this material. I also lead a workshop titled *Essentials for Sharing the Gospel with Oil*. These additions give this material "hands and feet," and hopefully demonstrate how to effectively share Biblical stories using all kinds of amazing fragrant plants.

What Is the Intended Readership for This Book?

I wrote this book for a variety of readers:

- Men and women who produce, market, or own an essential oil business
- School and Sunday School teachers, pastors, seminary students
- Essential oil hobbyists
- Medical professionals
- Gardeners
- Women's groups

- Book clubs
- Those taking an interest in wine, olive oil, and honey tasting
- Anyone desiring a better understanding of Hebrew covenant promises and their holy days found in Leviticus 23, and how plants and fragrances were essential in covenant worship
- Those who want to gain a better understanding of God's promises, especially where specific plants cropped up again and again in the Old and New Testament stories
- Anyone concerned about our environment and learning new ways to keep it health, as alternative suggestions are given for blending fragrant plant compounds when some of these plants are found threatened.

A special thank you for your encouragement, proof reading, theological, and English reviews, feedback, and suggestions:

Jimmy Cobb
Susan Booth
Eulonda Dreher
Cheryl Evans
Michael Hampton
Salt Jones
Lawson Lau
Alicja Mackiewicz
and
Wendy Meador

DETAILED TABLE OF CONTENTS

Chapters

1. **Ancient of Days, Light, and His Aromatic Bouquet**
   Fragrant offering of herbs
   Biblical references for herbs and the light of Creation
   Historical application of herbs
   Creation of days one, two, three and four
   The creation of edible herbs
   In three days

2. **Frankincense and the Table of the Bread of Presence**
   Fragrant offering of frankincense
   Biblical references for frankincense
   Historical application of frankincense
   On days five, six, and seven (the Sabbath)
   Original sin and eternal life
   Fictional thoughts about Adam and Eve
   More about the delicious deadly fruit
   Grain and the Altar of the Bread of Presence
   The wise men's gift of frankincense

3. **Olive Oil and Wine for the Bridegroom**
   Fragrant offering of oil and wine
   Biblical references for oil and wine
   Historical application of oil and wine
   Oil for the seven lamps on the lampstand
   The ten bridesmaids and the Bridegroom

4. **Acacia Wood for the Day of Atonement**
   Fragrant offering of acacia
   Biblical references for acacia wood
   Historical application of acacia wood
   The Tabernacle and the Ark of the Covenant
   Linen and the Day of Atonement
   The cross and the crown of thorns

5. Myrrh, Consecration, and the Altar of Burnt Offering
Fragrant offering of myrrh
Biblical references for myrrh
Historical application of myrrh
Myrrh in the holy anointing oil
Myrrh and the Altar of Burnt Offering
The Romans and myrrh at the cross

6. Cinnamon, Cassia, and Calamus in the Holy Anointing Oil
Fragrant offering of cinnamon
Biblical references for cinnamon
Historical application of cinnamon
Cinnamon and the bronze Basin
Jacob and Joseph lived – and died – in Egypt
Myrrh, aloes and spice
In three days and the resurrection

7. Mary Anoints Jesus with Spikenard
Fragrant offering of nard
Biblical references for nard
Historical application of nard
The Role of Women in Israel
Mary and the anointing of Jesus for His burial
Pentecost and the anointing of the disciples

8. Myrtle, Palm, and Willow for the Festival of the Booths
Fragrant offering of myrtle
Biblical references for myrtle and leafy woods
Historical application of myrtle and leafy woods
The Prophet Noah and the ark
Ezra and the inspiration for Sukkot
Jesus and His preparation of a room.

9. Hyssop for Cleansing and Purity
Fragrant offering of hyssop
Biblical references for hyssop
Historical application of hyssop

Hyssop's role in purification
Moses and the raising up of hyssop for Passover
Hyssop and its presence at the Cross

10. **Galbanum with Onycha, and Our Great High Priest**
    Fragrant offering of galbanum
    Biblical references for gall and onycha
    Historical application of bitter herbs and gall
    The Great High Priest and the Altar of Incense
    Jesus and his role as Great High Priest

11. **Cedarwood, Cypress, and Fir for the Temple**
    Fragrant offering of cedarwood
    Biblical references for cedarwood
    Historical application of cedarwood
    Cedarwood and its use in King Solomon's Temple
    Herod's Temple and Ezekiel's Temple
    The temple of God and our bodies

12. **Healing Leaves for the Nations**
    Fragrant offering of dew
    Biblical references for healing leaves
    Historical application of healing leaves
    The parable of the soils and the seed
    Aromatic seals and their ancient uses
    Brokenness and healing
    The Festival of Trumpets and the Day of the Lord

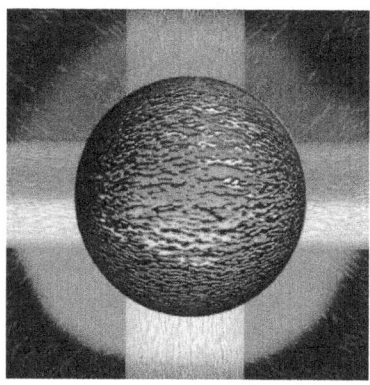

Chapter 1

The Ancient of Days, Light, and His Aromatic Bouquet

Make a fragrant offering of herbs

As you read through each chapter consider putting together a fragrant collection of plants, flowers and herbs. For this chapter I suggest making a bouquet of aromatic herbs using fresh lavender, thyme, rosemary, basil, mint, or many others.

Plant name: *Garni bouquet.* This chapter celebrates all aromatic plants and their benefits.

Oil extraction/characteristics: A very low percentage of all plants contain cells which produce oil sacks on their leaves. These are the plants which can be used to make essential oils. Some of these same plants are also used as aromatic herbs for perfumery, for our diet, or for medicinal purposes.

Flower petals can also be used to extract their fragrance in a process called *enfleurage*, which uses fats. The first record of this process was found on the Cuneiform tablets from Babylon which were written in 1200 BC. This is a very slow, expensive and time-consuming process. The Arabs, Egyptians, and East Asians all practiced perfumery in ancient times.

Aroma: Aromatherapists, perfumers and chefs use herbs for their fragrance, chemicals, oils, and flavorings. Fragrances can also be described by the plant's name, aroma, or their taste and smell. For example:

> anise, balsamic, bitter, camphor, citrus, conifer, dry, earthy, floral, fresh, fruity, green, grass-like, heady, herby, herbaceous, heavy, light, lemony, spicy, minty, musty, nutty, piney, powdery, rose-like, rich, sweet, sharp, smooth, turpentine-like, warm, woody, and weedy.

A satisfying way to refine our olfactory senses is to explore the plant life all around us, and then practice describing it. Sometimes the actual plants' chemicals are used to describe the aroma. For example "cineole," a constituent found in eucalyptus, has its own distinct aroma which may also be used to describe its fragrance.

Biblical references for the light of Creation

- In the beginning God created days one to four (Genesis 1:1-19). Throughout the Bible when God chose to interact with men or women, they frequently witnessed a bright light.
- Moses recorded that an angel of the Lord appeared to him from within the flames of a burning bush that somehow was not consumed. God asked him to return to Egypt and free the Israelites (Exodus 3:2).
- God provided a pillar of fire by night and a pillar of cloud by day *for forty years* for the Israelites in their desert wandering (Exodus 13:21; Joshua 5:6).
- King David, a musician, poet and a warrior, wrote that God had delivered him from death and kept his feet from stumbling, so that he could walk before God *"in the light of life"* (Psalm 56:13 ESV), and *"The unfolding of your words gives light;"* (Psalm 119:130 ESV).
- Over and over in the Bible, light is other-worldly. Isaiah spoke of a great light for those *"who walked in darkness have seen a great light"* (Isaiah 9:2 ESV).
- The LORD declared His Word is like fire (Jeremiah 23:29).

- At Jesus' birth the shepherds were witnessed angels and "*the glory of the Lord shone around them*" (Luke 2:9 ESV).
- Matthew wrote that when Mary Magdalene and the other Mary went to the tomb to finish anointing Jesus, an angel of the Lord appeared to them. He rolled away the large stone covering the entrance of the tomb and the women saw that the angel's "*appearance was like lightning*" (Matthew 28:3 ESV).
- When Peter's chains fell off in prison a light shone in his prison cell (Acts 12:7).
- Saul (who was later called Paul) was blinded by a great light as he was traveling to persecute the new Christian church (Acts 26:13).
- Paul wrote about *an unapproachable light,* which he also experienced (1 Timothy 6:16).
- Paul also wrote that every person's work shall be made known "*for the Day will disclose it*" (1 Corinthians 3:13 ESV).
- John, a disciple and a beloved friend of Jesus, wrote about his vision of an angel came from heaven and "*His face was like the sun*" (Revelation 10:1 ESV).

The true light that gives light to everyone was coming into the world. He was in the world, and though the world was made through him, the world did not recognize him (John 1:9-10 NIV).

• On the other hand, Satan "*disguises himself as an angel of light*" (2 Corinthians 11:14 ESV). Why would he do this? Because he knows how powerful light is, and how much the light draws us to it.

Historical application for herbs

As long as men and women have been on the planet, plants have been collected from the wild or cultivated, to sustain their diet and to use them for healing. Compounds in the form of teas, oils, tinctures, salves, or balms have been gathered and applied. Bundling specific herbs together into a poultice and placing them on a wound was thought to pull out infection from the body and to inhibit inflammation which then reduced pain.

- The prophet Isaiah gave instructions to King Hezekiah's servants to press figs into a lump and when they applied it to King Hezekiah's boil, he recovered (2 Kings 20:7).
- Elisha put flour in a pot to diffuse poison in a toxic stew (2 Kings 4:39-41).
- Rachel and Leah had a dispute over mandrake plants which may have been thought to have fertility properties (Genesis 30:14-17).
- Job compared God's ability to form the sea to like making *"a pot of ointment"* (Job 41:31).

Eating specific herbal plants has historically been used to help restore balance when experiencing pain, gastronomical discomfort, or any kind of illness. Aromatic plant material has also been used for inhalation to recover one's vitality after an emotional or physical trauma, or for respiratory distress from disease.

When our Creator made the heavens and the earth, He interconnected the health of the planet to the health of all living beings. The cells in our body are sustained by plant fibers, fluids, vitamins, minerals, and the compounds that make up plants. Plants produce oxygen that fills our lungs and sustains animal life. In turn we produce carbon dioxide which supports plant life.

Can we live without plants? Even if this were possible, I doubt whether we would want to live without them, because they stimulate our senses and give us such enjoyment as we discover and appreciate each variety, design, color, taste, and aroma. We have always been a part of God's Garden, and the Garden was designed to be a part of us.

Since I did not choose specific plants for this chapter, I want to comment on the processes of blending plants for the purpose of making a bouquet, for seasoning food, and for blending aromatic fragrances.

The French word *garni* bouquet means garnished bouquet. Fresh garden herbs like oregano, thyme, basil, lavender, and some fruits can all be used to make a soup stock or to flavor dishes. Tying up or bundling herbs with string or plant leaves can be used for cooking meats and vegetables. This releases flavors and aromas and enhances any meal. One mark of a good cook is that he or she has learned how to use seasoning well.

In 1857 a Frenchman named Septimus Piesse[i], wrote *The Art of Perfumery.* He was a chemist and a perfumer who described plant fragrances as having notes like music. He described top, middle, and base note fragrances. Rose, clove, and cinnamon are base notes, lavender and marjoram are middle notes, and fennel, tarragon and thyme are top notes. Many times perfumers blend top, middle, and base notes because they believe these types of fragrances complement each other in ways that similar notes cannot.

Every continent and country on the earth has been blessed with a unique array of fragrances from its own indigenous plant life: cinnamon from India or southeast Asia; bay from Asia Minor; clove from Indonesia; mandarin orange from China; clary sage from Russia; cardamom from Sri Lanka; and so many others.

Some of the loveliest blends of EOs are those which have been grown in opposite corners of the earth or are separated by a great geographical distance. For example, one of my favorite blends is eucalyptus and lavender. *Eucalyptus globulus* from Australia with its musty, green, woody, refreshing camphor, and *cineole* of eucalyptus combined with *Lavandula angustifolia* from Europe with its fresh, sweet, floral, refreshing, herbaceous, balsamic-woody fragrance creates an amazing aromatic blend.

The earth was – and is – adorned with a living, aromatic bouquet.

Creation of days one, two, three, and four

Essence of Day

In the beginning the earth was without form and empty and the waters covered the surface of the Earth.

On day one God created light. The Bible describes that there was evening and morning on the first day, that God completed the creation of our heaven and earth in six days, and then He rested on the seventh day.

How do these Scriptures define a "day?" For the ancient Hebrew, a day began at sunset ended at the next sunset. Each holy day celebration also began at sunset.

On day one of Creation God said, "Let there be light" (Genesis 1:3). Was this light of the same spectrum of light we are familiar with that we now know as day light or "white light"? We simply do not know the scientific specifics about the light of Creation. The scientific community is just now beginning to understand our own planet's sunlight.

Using quantum mechanics, scientists recently discovered what we perceive as day light is perplexing because it behaves as a wave and a particle. For centuries, scientists hotly debated the question, "Is light a wave or a particle?" In 2015 Ecole Polytechnique Fédérale de Lausanne[ii] published an article that demonstrates light is both!

Science and the Bible do not oppose each other if one believes that the Creator set all things in motion, including the rules of the universe. In fact, the only way science can accomplish anything is because the universe operates according to His design and physical laws.

The next 3 days of creation were busy ones for God. On day two He separated the water from the sky. On day three He separated dry ground from the seas and created plants. On day four He created the sun, moon, and stars. The Holy Bible has a powerful story to tell about the creative energy of God, an energy with which he has imbued us as beings made in His image.

Going back to day three, God spoke and plants emerged, with their energy-collecting cells called chloroplasts, and they began to interact with the light of creation.

When the creation of earth was complete, I can only imagine the visual beauty and the aromatic fragrances released from such wonders as:

- the pristine cedars of Lebanon in their full crown and glory;
- the amazing giant cypress sequoias of California;
- the Tianshan Xueling spruce forest of China;
- the Boreal forest of Russia;
- the rainforest of Brazil;
- the chapel oaks of the Netherlands and Europe;
- the Montezuma cypress of Mexico;
- the sandalwood trees of India;
- the olive trees from Crete, Greece, Israel, Italy and Spain;
- the mahogany of Australia;
- the Sycamore fig of Africa;
- and so many others that still survive, and sadly some that did not.

Day three, would have been nothing like we have ever experienced. At its completion, generous amounts of fragrant plant volatiles and pheromones would have been released, creating their own atmosphere for life.

God created plants to serve all the creatures of the earth. This includes mankind, as we participated in the marvelous exchange of carbon dioxide for oxygen. In a very real sense, plants gave (and continues to give) the breath of life to all peoples of every nation on earth.

A very small percentage of plants grow special cells called trichomes, which are microscopic oil sacks. These cells protect the plant from severe hot and cold temperatures, diseases, molds, fungi, and insects. Many of these plants are aromatic and are used to make essential oils or medicinal oils.

Even in today's advancing scientific community the exact process of how plants create oil is not completely understood.[iii] There is still a lot we do not understand about the earth, creation, and the *Ancient of Days,* our Creator God

(Daniel 7:9). Science is at its best when it approaches our complex creation with humility and questions rather than arrogance and proclamations.

Jesus told Nicodemus, who was a Hebrew priest, about being "born again," but Nicodemus did not understand how he as a grown man could *be* born again. We may agree we need to be reborn in our heart, mind, and soul; but do we understand exactly how we are being, or might be transformed? Jesus asks us to learn from the things that surround us in creation, in order to get a glimpse of the eternal things which we cannot see with our eyes:

> *I have spoken to you of earthly things and you do not believe; how then will you believe if I speak of heavenly things? (John 3:12 NIV).*

As we gaze into the heavens and attempt to fathom the extent of all creation, our minds can barely comprehend eternity and the role we were in which we were created to take part. Even with the most powerful telescopes known to man, we still only see a fraction of what has been created.

Mankind's original design and purpose described in Genesis was to have dominion over the earth. Having control or authority over the earth still remains a great challenge for us as we struggle to cope with everyday issues like environmental changes, social injustice of all kinds, technological advancements, national security, and our own personal issues with everyday life. Paul wrote:

> *For his eternal power and divine nature, have been clearly perceived ever since the creation of the world (Romans 1:20 ESV).*

The ancient Israelites understood that God ordered all things, and He is sovereign over all. There was darkness, but God separated the darkness from the light. In the same way, He can separate the darkness from the light in each one of us.

The creation of edible herbs

Every week the Israelites celebrated the completion of creation by observing the seventh day, or *Shabbat* (Sabbath), as sacred. It was to be set apart and to be remembered as holy. They organized their calendar year along God's lines, by establishing holy days from typical days. When each holy day began, they recited an ancient blessing called *Havdalah,* which is a prayer of thanksgiving. Interestingly enough a portion of this prayer includes a blessing for their fragrant seasonings. "*Remember the Sabbath day, to keep it holy*" (Exodus 20:8 ESV).

At some point in the Israelites" history, they also adopted the use of three items to mark *Havdalah*: the lighting of two candles or oil lamps, the drinking of wine, and the inhaling of a box of sweet-smelling spices as a reminder of the fragrance of *Shabbat*, so that they might retain a fragrant memory of His rest throughout their coming week. We can also follow in the path of the ancient Israelites by using fragrance to remind us of God's promises!

Today the western world is a fusion of cultures similar to that in the Middle East during the time of Jesus. There was Roman occupation of Israel when Caesar and King Herod were in charge. Roman law could and would overrule the Hebraic law, which was as you might expect was greatly resented by Israel (John 11:49-50).

The Israelites practiced dietary and social restrictions which separated clean from unclean. This clashed in almost every way with Roman polytheism, diet, culture, social, and religious practices. This is not unlike the cultural conflicts we have today in the western world.

Greek, Palestinian, Persian, Arab, Babylonian, Egyptian, and others coexisted and blended through marriage on Israel's borders. There was also influence from Asia, which filtered in through the Grain Roads. Although fragrant plants harvested and collected for Jerusalem's temple worship were also valued by others in the area, they did not use them for the same religious purpose.

Jesus, who is called "Christ" (the anointed One[1]), instructed the disciples that the tabernacle and the temple were temporary. Paul added that they were designed to be a *copy and a shadow of heavenly things,* but this has become increasingly difficult for us to fully comprehend (Hebrews 8:5).

Due to our own cultural filters and the passage of time, we may never fully grasp all of the ways in which the people in the Holy Lands viewed the uses of plants for medical or religious purposes, but one thing is certain: Aromatic herbs in the ancient world were highly valued, and were a vital component of their lives.

During the Passover celebrations the markets in Jerusalem would have been full of spices. They would have been packed with merchants and travelers. Israelites who lived outside of Jerusalem would travel in for this and other annual holy days.

If followers of the faith traveled from very far, they would bring dried spices, dates, and raisins so they could also present a tithe to the temple (Leviticus 27:30; Nehemiah 10:37). According to the law, tithes were to be ten percent of their total harvest. Any excess goods they had could have been sold in the marketplace to help pay for their expenses.

The Levite priests lived on the food offerings presented to the temple by the people, and some of the offerings were prepared and used for the incense, lamps, and the anointing oil which were part of the sacraments used for worship.

---

[1] "Messiah" has the same connotation as "Christ" and "Anointed One."

According to the laws God gave Moses, the tithe was the Levite priests' inheritance, because they did not inherit land like the other eleven tribes of Israel (Deuteronomy 14:22-29; 18:1-2). It appears that the Levite's themselves also participated in giving a tithe – a tithe on the people's tithe!

Jesus, who was born an Israelite and raised in this religious tradition, warned the teachers of the law and the scribes that they were hypocritical when they gave a tenth of their mint, dill, and cumin, but were not interested in justice, mercy, and faithfulness (Matthew 23:23). He wasn't implying that the spices weren't valuable. On the contrary, he was comparing these valuable fragrant herbs with the yet more valuable spiritual possessions.

Before the Sabbath, women in Israel would have been busy preparing a special dish with *tavlin,* which means "spice".[2] This dish had a blend of extra salt, pepper, and spices that was eaten on the Sabbath day. Why cook before the Sabbath? Moses' covenant law for the Sabbath Day was very specific; no one was permitted to work. This included making a flame or cooking food. The extra spices were added in part to keep the food from going rancid before they could eat it the following day. We still use many of these spices for cooking because of their flavors, but at one time they were also valued for their antibacterial and antifungal properties that prevent the food from growing harmful bacteria.

Before modern refrigeration, spice (along with extra salt) was critical to keep food from going bad. Why? Because these meals might sit for hours before they were consumed. Spices had a crucial value that we no longer consider, but the ancients had to rely on for food and spice for medication. This is also one of the reasons why Europeans searched the world for a passage to the spice islands of Southeast Asia and instead discovered North America. North American ginger was also grown and used by its indigenous people. It was so highly

---

[2] Hebrew Conjugation Tables, Search tavlin, https://www.pealim.com/dict/5555-tavlin/

valued as a medicine it was exported and traded by the early settlers.

The spice and grain trade opened up shipping routes through oceans and into the Bible lands of the Middle East. Highly traveled caravan routes called the "Grain Roads" were used to transport goods in and out of Jerusalem. Later these roads would be used by the disciples to carry the Good News out of Jerusalem. Later still they became known as the Spice Roads which were used into the 15th century.

Caraway, dill, fennel, ginger, mint, mustard seed, sesame, safflower, and thyme are herbs that were used in ancient Israel, and with which most westerners are still familiar with today (Matthew 13:31). Not all of these spices are found in the Bible; some are mentioned in the Babylonian Talmud[3] the Israelites wrote during their time in captivity.

China, Egypt, Persia, and India also kept records of the spices they valued. *Cardamom* is one of the oldest spices recorded for its use in Ayurvedic medicine from India and Chinese medicine.[iv] Cardamom with lots of sugar is still used to flavor coffee in Amman, Jordan and the Middle East. It gives the coffee a warm, spicy, and cineole (eucalyptus) like flavor and odor.

There were also *capers* which are briny, tangy, and lemony; *Cumin,* which is spicy, nutty, earthy, with a bitter lemon undertone; and *Rue* or *ruta graveolens*, a citrus plant historically used for medicinal purposes and to flavor dishes (Luke 11:42). Rue has a bitter taste, but the blossoms and shoots are considered to be the most valuable part of the plant for eating. Dried rue is used for tea.[v]

Saffron is mentioned in the Bible (Song of Solomon 4:14). Most of us in the West do not have much experience cooking

---

[3] Essentially an ancient commentary on the Scriptures written by the Hebrew's during their captivity in Babylon.

with *saffron,* which is the stamen of a crocus flower named *crocus sativus.* I savored a rice dish made with high quality saffron called tahchin, that was prepared by an Iranian woman in Toronto. It was flavorful, delicate, sweet, and quite unique. When asked by our host to describe its flavor, I could not find the words.

Isn't it interesting that we might be unsuccessful in knowing or finding a word which describes a fragrance or flavor, because it is nothing like we have ever experienced or sensed before? You might experience tastes or smells like this crocus, which would make it *saffron-like.* We might also consider the fragrance of saffron so heavenly we just do not have the vocabulary to describe it yet. Most saffron sold in the west has lost its flavor, so I have never had any success in reproducing this dish. Saffron is also marketed as a supplement for mood support, which causes me to wonder if this plant is sustainable, and who is able to grow that much Saffron?

Every spice blend is distinct to the one cooking. Geographical areas seem to develop their own preferences. There is also a possibility that our bodies prefer flavorings because of a nutritional or physical need or craving. There was and is a spice blend in the Middle East called *savory (zaatar in Arabic) Savory* is a blend that sometimes adds *Lavandula stoechas L.,* a type of plant that grew and grows as a wild shrub in the Middle East. It is similar to our modern-day lavender. Savory is often blended with thyme, hyssop, and sumac which is still a popular flavor in the Middle East among Arab and Jewish cooks. Sumac can be used in place of lemon for flavor. There are reasons to believe Lavandula may have also been exported to Spain and then France. Some blends of savory have similarities to a spice blend from France named *Herbes de Provence,* a blend that is sometimes also made with lavender.

The Lord will be our light

Essence of Day

The Bible describes a *"Kingdom of Light,"* when there will be no need for light from the sun or moon because *God* will be our light (Colossians 1:12). As you may recall, in the creation account of Genesis plants were created on day three, which was *before* the creation of the heavenly bodies, the sun, and the moon (Genesis 1:13).

It is amazing to think about how this might have been, as we come to realize how little we know about the Creator of Day, apart from what we know about His only Son, Jesus.

Isaiah, John and Peter also wrote that one day there will be a new heaven and a new earth. John wrote there will be no need for light from the sun, moon, or stars because God is and will continue to be our sustaining light. How awesome is that?!

> *And night will be no more. They will need no light of lamp or sun, for the Lord God will be their light* (Revelation 22:5 ESV).

Life would not exist without light, but is this light of Creation the same light we perceive as sunlight? The human eye can only detect white light, but there are other spectrums of light our eyes cannot detect; for example, red or infrared light, and at the other end of the spectrum, blue-violet (UV) light. The earth's atmosphere blocks most of the UV light, but some of its operation helps regulate our wake-sleep cycle and our ability to stay alert. It also affects our cognition, memory, and emotional health. But we could have too much of a good thing: If all of the blue light got through the atmosphere, we could not survive.

Herb farmers have discovered that if they grow plants under artificial UV lights it decreases pathogens both on the plants and in the water they absorb. The added stress the UV light places on the plants encourages them to expand the size of their trichome cells, which drives them to produce more oil to protect the plant. This is similar to the way the Word of God adds stress to our soul, which causes us to struggle so that we may begin to receive more and more of the anointing of the Spirit.

In the Garden of Eden, God gave Adam and Eve His blessing and all was good. After their fall, their having dominion over the earth came with new difficulties. Today science is continually uncovering the various negative impacts that humans are having on the environment. These may even become a challenge to our own lives as plants and animals are being stressed to levels never experienced on earth before.

Men and women also need forgiveness for the sins they have committed against the earth. I cannot begin to list all of the harm done to the earth's plants and animals, but I have taken note that the aromatic plants and trees in this study, currently harvested for their essential oils, are at risk. We should never take the health of our earth for granted. We all need to do our part to protect plants, our atmosphere and the animals that bring balance and harmony to the earth's ecosystem. This includes finding substitutes for essential oils made from plants that are endangered.

We need to become better caretakers and educators of the earth and do our best to keep her vital and healthy, even when our ultimate hope is in a new heaven and new earth (Isaiah 66:22; Daniel 7; 2 Peter 3; 1 John 4:17; Revelation 21:1).

To discover the sustainability of the plant in question, you can search the *Redlist.com*, or the United States Department of Agriculture, also keeps a list. To keep current on the state of these and other aromatic plants, renew your searches from time to time. Why? Because plant propagation can change for the better or worse. Continue to check the condition of the plant in question annually. Here is an update on some of the threatened plants in this study:

1. Olive Oil: *Olea europaea subsp. cerasiformis* (NT); near threatened.

2. Frankincense (NT); near threatened.
3. *Santalum album* or Sandalwood (VU); vulnerable.
4. *Aquilaria malaccensis* or Agarwood *(CE);* critically endangered species.
5. *Cedrus libani* or Cedar of Lebanon (VU); vulnerable.
6. *Cedrus atlantica* or Cedarwood Atlas (TS); threatened species 2013.
7. *Nardostachys jatamansi* or Spikenard/Nard (CR); critically endangered species.

When I see a bouquet and take in its fragrance, I am reminded of a wonderful parallel: that the Creator of Day gave life to the plants on day three, and the crucified Christ rose from the dead, on day three. I don't believe that this is a coincidence, because from the beginning of creation El-Shaddai—God Almighty—has had this in His grand design.

$$\approx A\Omega \approx$$

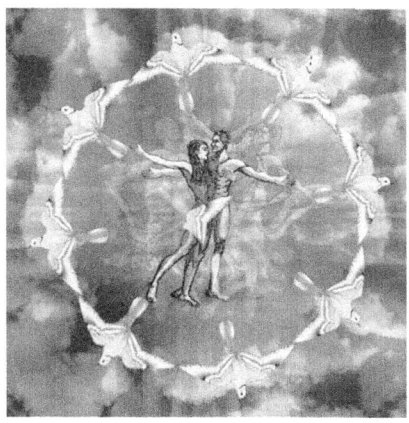

Chapter 2

Frankincense and the Table of the Bread of Presence

The fragrant offering of frankincense

For this chapter I suggest making your own fragrant offering by setting a table with raw pine resin using dried orange - lemon or lime peel, or fresh oranges and pine branches for a table centerpiece. Any of these fragrances may also be used in a diffuser.

Substitute: Frankincense is on the Red List[vi] as near threatened (NT). To duplicate the fragrance of frankincense, create a blend of Cedarwood virginia or pine essential oil with a hint of lime or lemon 3/1 ratio. Although the chemical constituents are different, the aroma is very similar.

Plant name: Frankincense, *Boswellia sacra* or Olibanum, Boswellia, from the Latin root meaning *oleum libani, (oil of Lebanon)*. Family: *Burseraceae*. Mostly from Oman, Yemen and southern Saudi Arabia, but other subspecies are from Somalia, Ethiopia and western India.

Oil extraction/characteristics: Steam distillation is used to separate the essential oils from dried and crushed tree resin. Frankincense essential oil is a mobile or liquid essential oil which is pale, yellow-green-to amber. A white sap is released from the Boswellia tree which dries and hardens into a tea-colored resin that can be ground, heated in oil, boiled in water, distilled by steam, or ground and burned in its raw form.

The origins of the word "perfume" come from the Latin words *"per fumus,"* which means through the smoke (referring to the release of the fragrance by burning).

The Israelites could have also burned frankincense for their own personal use, which is why the people were warned by Moses not to replicate the recipe for the holy incense or they would be cut off from Israel (Exodus 30:38). The priests most likely kept the exact details for making the holy incense and holy anointing oil a secret, but my research on plant extracts leads me to believe that most of this would have been common knowledge for those who could afford to purchase them or collect the components.

Aroma: My bottle of frankincense essential oil has an aroma similar to that of pine wood with a hint of turpentine, which makes it terpene-like, and a fruity lift of lime, or lemon.

Emotional benefits: Frankincense can be used to alleviate an accumulation of stress and irritability, restlessness, and insomnia. [vii] Cedarwood oil and white fir are also sedatives and can be helpful for chronic conditions of anxiety and nervous tension.[viii]

Biblical references for frankincense

- Aromatic tree resins were found in the land of Havilah, or the Garden of Eden (Genesis 2:11-12).
- As we have seen frankincense was included in the recipe for the holy incense (Exodus 30:34).
- Frankincense was placed on the Table of the Bread of Presence and was included in the priestly duties in the temple when after it

was linked to the covenant promises God made to Israel (Leviticus 2:1).
- Frankincense was presented for a sin offering (Leviticus 5:11).
- Frankincense was presented to Jesus by the wise men.
- We're told that the merchants of the earth shall weep and not be able to find precious wood, citrus wood, ivory, frankincense and many other items including *"souls of men"* (Revelation 18:12-13). Interesting that precious natural chemical compounds like aromas are compared to the souls of men.

Historical application of frankincense

When Adam and Eve went against God's will, they were driven out of the Garden of Eden by an angel who guarded the way so they could not return. This is the first time in the Bible we find an angel who appeared as a messenger or warrior.

They were banished from the safety of the garden as an otherworldly creature guarded the way back to the garden. This would have certainly caused a lot of stress, anxiety, regret and shame for Adam and Eve. The Scriptures go on to disclose that God did not abandon Adam and Eve, but instead continued to desire and pursue a relationship with them, just like He does with us.

One of the things that makes the Hebraic Bible so interesting to read is that people's mistakes as well as their achievements were recorded. It is rare to find this kind of transparency in the historic documents of other nations.

Some of Israelites' sins were against God and other sins were against each other, but all of them had consequences for them individually and as a nation. However, God promised that if they would live by His covenant plan, He would be with them no matter what. God did this by making a pattern of His plan in the design and function of the tabernacle. The duties that were carried out by the priests in their daily exercises, included the use of fragrant plants, and burnt offerings as a reflection of Heavenly things.

King David wrote that we are fearfully and wonderfully made (Psalm 139:14). Our ability to perceive, enjoy or dislike a fragrance is somehow both fearful and wonderful and may serve a greater purpose than we fully comprehend. Dried resin from the Boswellia tree in its natural state is sometimes called tears because of the shape it takes when it drips off the tree to the ground and hardens. How might our tears reflect how our Creator made us in His image? Could they also represent His tears?

On days five, six, and seven (the Sabbath)

On day five of creation, God filled the sky and the seas with every living creature that flies and swims. This included amazing creatures like whales, which are air-breathing mammals who live under water! Surprisingly Sperm Whales produce a waxy substance called ambergris in their digestive tracts that has been used as a fixative by perfumers for centuries.

On day six of creation, God created the animals that would live on the land. His work culminated with the creation of Adam and Eve. Throughout God's description of His work, He makes it plain that human beings are a completely separate creation, the only living beings made in God's own image.

On the seventh day of creation, God rested from all the work He had done in creation (Genesis 1:11-19; 2:15-17). In the Hebraic account of creation the seventh day is described as "separate" or "holy." The Hebraic word *vyenafesh or wayyinnaphesh* transliterated for "rest" can mean many things depending on its usage. It can mean to *ensoul*[ix], to have *breath*, a *pleasing fragrance*, an *appetite*, a *passion*, or a *joy* that *yearns* in our *inner soul*.[x] Another word derived from the Hebrew word for "rest" is the word *nepesh*, which means to be alive or to *breathe* as a *living soul*.[xi] So on the Sabbath, God rested His living soul. We also have the opportunity to follow His example and rest in Him every seven days. For the Israelites this began Friday at sunset and went to Saturday at sunset. The important thing is that we set aside time to rest and turn our senses toward a full day of experiencing our Creator God.

Adam and Eve lived in the Garden of Eden, which was also known as the land of Havilah. Scholars believe that Havilah was located near the junction of the Tigris and the Euphrates Rivers where aromatic resins were also found. These aromatic resins likely included frankincense.

Adam and Eve would have had an extraordinary relationship in the garden with their Creator God. We're told that they walked with God in the "cool of the evening." Wouldn't you love to go out on that kind of walk?! (Genesis 3:8)

However, the book of Genesis also recorded that there were two trees in the center of the garden. One was called the tree of life and the other the tree of knowledge of good and evil. God forbid Adam or Eve to touch or eat fruit from the tree of the knowledge of good and evil, and gave them a stern warning that if they ate it, they would die.

We know from this account in Genesis God created men and women to have the freedom to act outside of His perfect will. He encouraged them to eat the fruit from every other tree in the garden except for the tree of knowledge in the center of the garden. Why did He do this? This was for their own protection, but because God is all knowing He knew they could eventually fail Him. From this account in the Bible, we understand right from the beginning God's desire was for Adam and Eve to choose the fruit of life not death. God's original design was for us to inherit and possess an everlasting life.

Original sin and eternal life

Most of us fail to understand why evil was allowed to exist in the garden at all. Why would God allow the entrance of an evil being who masqueraded as good? This malicious serpent was able to persuade Eve to go against the Creator's will and to take fruit from the only forbidden tree. She invited Adam to join her, and he did. Because of their actions, they both drastically fell from the relationship they had with God (Genesis 2-3; 3:1-24; Isaiah 14:13-15)?

God created Adam and Eve with the ability to make their own decisions as they experienced and interacted with the created world around them. The Creator fashioned our brains to perceive sight, sound, touch, smell, taste, and the desire to investigate all that He created.

Amazingly, men and women are able to distinguish over 10,000 different plant fragrances. These range from desirable to unpleasant with only subtle differences to the molecular structure in each of these plant chemicals. The part of our brain responsible for interpreting what is happening around us in our environment us called the limbic system.

When we breathe, air particles called odorants they connect with special receptor cells inside our nose, in a process called chemoreception or olfaction.[xii] Then the limbic system filters this information and influences our motivation, memory, learning, and our ability to stay alert or disengage. All of this is interconnected with the part of our brain which is tied into our sense of smell. The limbic system is also involved in making choices and remembering those outcomes.[xiii]

Everything Adam and Eve needed was right there in the garden to nourish and refresh them. No doubt they would have had preferences for food and aromas like we do. They would have been able to remember what they preferred in the form of textures, colors, tastes, and smells. There is no mention of eating meat, apparently because the garden appeared to sustain them without it.

Adam and Eve had a symbiotic relationship with all animals, plants, and with their Creator God in the Garden. Whatever Adam did in the garden, it gave back and vice versa. A perfect life, but one that came with a single command: do not eat from the tree of knowledge of good and evil or *"you shall die"* (Genesis 2:17).

Fictional thoughts about Adam and Eve

I can imagine the fruit with which Eve was tempted with was most like a peach. The peach tree or *Prunus persica* is a tree from the *Rosaceae* family of plants. After the serpent was able to persuade Eve to investigate the peach (or whatever fruit is was), she no doubt would have considered it quite beautiful to contemplate. Its white vellus hairs which reflect light over the yellow orange to dark red shades on its skin give it a unique peach color and texture.

With the serpent masquerading as a friend, telling her she could become wise, knowing good and evil like God, Eve investigated it further and picked the fruit (Genesis 3:6). The peach may have felt warm, soft, and heavy in her hand as this hydrating fruit is mostly water. She may have pressed the warm, velvety fruit up against her upper lip and nose to take in its honey, almond, rose-like floral fragrance. Then by pressing her thumb nail through its subtle skin near the dimple made by its stem she may have cut around its circumference following its suture line, and with a bit of a twist she could have split the fruit in half. There she would have seen a flat shaped seed striped and pierced with indentations. As Eve brought the peach to her lips, the sweet honey-like nectar that had dampened her fingertips would have touched her taste buds on the end of her tongue, which would have suddenly stimulated her salivary glands.

When Eve saw the fruit was good for eating, God's instructions, that she should not eat, must have quickly faded into the back of her mind as she became beguiled by the deceiver. Eve may have acted on her predispositions and on her desire for a God-like wisdom, instead of keeping the instructions her Creator had given her. Maybe in Adam's attempt to please Eve, or because his desire to worship the created (Eve) was greater than it was for His Creator, he also ate the fruit.

More about the delicious, deadly fruit

The meat inside of each peach seed contains a chemical called cyanide, which in very small amounts is highly toxic. Cyanide is just as deadly as the decision Eve and Adam made when the seed of sin and death had been allowed to take root in their life. Their sin had consequences just as God had warned, but Adonai, their LORD and Master would never force them to serve Him. Eve had been deceived by a lesser authority, who was and still is permitted to imitate the greater One for the time being. It is written that Adam would now rule over Eve. Does this mean that they had been equal? Was this because Eve let go of God as the only true authority over her life? (Genesis 3:16)

Adam and Eve were driven out of the garden so they could not return and eat from the tree of eternal life. Cherubim (supper angels) were placed outside the garden to guard it (Genesis 3:24). Cherubim were fearsome warrior-like creatures first written about here, but who continue to appear throughout the Bible.

Why was evil allowed to co-exist in the garden? Why was it allowed to trick Eve into eating the fruit? These are the age-old questions each generation still asks. Our Creator God simply will not impose His will to gain our devotion. He wants us to recognize Him and give ourselves wholly, sincerely, and freely to Him.

Sadly, it is recorded that Adam and Eve's actions also affected the environment, and the land became cursed with thistles and thorns. Now they would have to labor to grow crops for their food, where before the garden bloomed and produced food for them on its own. Worst of all, their bodies like our own, would eventually expire in a physical death.

The serpent's lie to Eve in the garden, when he said, *"you will not surely die"* (Genesis 3:4 ESV), was also partly true only because of God's grace. As Adam's and Eve's physical bodies became subjected to time, in a definite order of death and decay, their eternal soul, or essence would remain like a fragrant vapor belonging and returning to their Creator God.

> *For the creation was subjected to futility, not willingly, but because of him who subjected it, in the hope that the creation itself will be set free from its bondage to corruption and obtain the freedom of the glory of the children of God. For we know that the whole creation has been groaning together in the pains of childbirth until now. And not only the creation but we ourselves who have the first fruits of the Spirit, groan inwardly as we wait eagerly for the redemption of our bodies* (Romans 8:20-23 ESV).

Sometime after Adam and Eve were driven out of the garden, they rediscovered aromatic resins similar to what had been in the land of Havilah (Genesis 2:12). They discovered these resins were abundant and useful. When they burned them on an open fire, they released their fragrance. This may have even help them relax and decrease their nervous tension after their traumatic fall.

When they boiled the plants' resin, they may have discovered the steam which was released helped ease respiratory distress. When they mixed it with an oil and applied it to their skin, they noticed it helped heal abrasions and ulcers. Frankincense and myrrh are both aromatic resins which are reported to help people feel relaxed and calm when they are under stress.[xiv]

Adam and Eve would have been greatly distressed and full of grief at the loss of the close relationship they had with God in the garden, a place where He had provided for them and communicated with them face to face. Now they were unsure about their environment and even their own safety. They may have burned frankincense to God as an offering in their desire to have His forgiveness and as a way to continue to acknowledge His presence. Our all-knowing God must have known that men and women could fail Him, but He would still pursue them, and He had another way to return them to Himself.

It is written that God Himself made clothing from animal skins to cover Adam and Eve because of the shame they experienced in their nakedness (Genesis 3:10; 21). This is the first time in Scripture we note the death of an animal because of sin. By clothing them, He gave them hope.

> *For I know the plans I have for you," declares the Lord, "plans to prosper you and not to harm you, plans to give you hope and a future* (Jeremiah 29:11 NIV).

Grain and the Altar of the Bread of Presence

After the fall, Adam and Eve had to work for their food by preparing the soil, planting seeds, pulling weeds, and harvesting crops, all of which became central for their survival. Separating the wheat from its chaff with its hard-outer cover and grinding grains into an edible flour became critical for their communities. This would have taken place around a threshing floor as their community acknowledged that God had provided another year's harvest for them.

Hunger was a big problem in the ancient world as droughts, plagues, and locusts impacted them on a regular basis. People relied on grains for sustenance when meat or vegetables were not available. Bread and olive oil were a common and satisfying staple for many. The people of the Bible lands planted what we call ancient grains which have been mentioned in the book of Ezekiel: wheat, barley, beans, lentils, millet, emmer, and spelt (Ezekiel 4:9). Bread had become a strong symbol of God's provision for ancient men and women. Why? Because its abundance was life and its scarcity could mean their death.

Generations after Adam and Eve, the Bible introduces us to Abraham and Sarah. God called Abraham (then known as Abram) out of the City of Ur or Chaldea south of the Euphrates and led him into Canaan. After God had delivered Abram from his enemies in battle, Melchizedek, the Most-High Priest and the King of Salem (King of Peace), came to Abram with bread and wine, and Abram gave the King ten percent of all he had (Genesis 14:18). Then God made a covenant with Abram and changed his name to Abraham.

The outward sign of this covenant was for every male child born to Abraham to be circumcised (Genesis 17:5-11). Abraham had two sons. His oldest son, Ishmael, was born to Hagar, his wife Sarah's handmaid, who Sarah had given to Abraham because she herself was barren. Abraham's other son, Isaac, was born to Sarah, incredibly after she was in her 90's!

Abraham circumcised Ishmael, and he became the father of the great Arab nations, but it was Isaac who would keep the covenant God made with Abraham so there would be no doubt that God intervened for them while Sarah was barren and way beyond her childbearing years. Isaac became the father of Jacob who became known as *"Israel"* (Genesis 35:10).

Jacob had two wives, Leah and Rachel. He became the father of 12 sons, who in time became the 12 tribes of Israel. Leah had 10 of those sons, and Rachel, Jacob's first and only true love, had two other sons, whom she named Joseph and Benjamin. Jacob favored Joseph, which caused his brothers to become jealous. His brother eventually sold Joseph into slavery when a caravan loaded with spices passed by on its way into Egypt.

This is interesting because we know from this passage that there were caravan routes for trading spices in the desert even this far back in Israel's history.

Essence of Day

The brothers lied and told their father Joseph had been eaten by a wild animal so he would not look for him (Genesis 37). Years later because of a famine in Canaan, Jacob, with his other eleven sons and their families were forced to go down to Egypt where there was enough grain in storage it would allow them to survive. In Egypt they rediscovered Joseph who through a series of miraculous interventions by God served in a high government position (Exodus 39:5). Joseph received his brothers and provided a way for them to stay in Egypt. Years later the Israelites became captive and were forced into slavery by future Pharaohs (Exodus 6:5).

Four generations later, Moses was born in Egypt. He was from the tribe of Levi, the third son of Jacob. Moses was the greatest prophet in Israel but he wrote that there would be an even greater prophet in the future of Israel and that they should be careful to hear and follow (Deuteronomy 18:15).

When Moses was about 80 years of age, he encountered God at a burning bush on Mt. Sinai. This is where God promised to help him return to Egypt to free the Israelites. With God's help, Moses led the twelve tribes out of their bondage. When he returned to Mount Sinai with the Israelites, God made another promise to Moses and the Israelites that if they would keep His covenant laws, they would become a chosen people, "*a kingdom of priests and a holy nation*" (Exodus 19:6 ESV).

During this time God provided manna for them to eat because there was not enough food in the desert. Manna would appear or settle on the ground in the mornings just like the dew and it looked like coriander seed (Numbers 11:7-9). Every morning the Israelites collected the manna and shaped it into cakes that looked like unleavened bread. God provided this wondrous food for them day by day as they wandered in the desert for 40 years.

God also gave Moses directions on how to build and worship in the tabernacle, which means "*a place to meet God.*" This included the design of six altars with all their utensils and the requirements for the daily work of the priests. God also instituted covenant laws to include a number of festivals to be observed annually (Leviticus 23).

Some of these requirements for offerings included frankincense along with wheat flour or kernels of grain. Both forms of grain were acceptable as first fruit offerings for the tabernacle. The wheat offering was accepted only if it had salt, olive oil, and frankincense placed with it. Pure frankincense resin in its raw form (tears) were also placed beside the twelve loaves of unleavened bread on the Altar of the Bread of Presence inside the tabernacle.

The bread on this table represented the unity of the twelve tribes. The priests would eat it as an act of worship to God, to acknowledge that He was present "in person." This altar was a table made from acacia wood and covered with gold and it had solid gold plates, bowls, and pitchers (Exodus 25:23-30). The wheat used to make unleavened bread for this table was to be ground into the finest flour. The priests cooked this bread as a fragrant offering in a pan on top of the Altar of Burnt Offering which was actually an open grill. The dough may have been scored, striped or pierced through to ensure that it cooked evenly, and prevent it from bubbling and deforming on a hot griddle. Every Sabbath Day the priests replaced the bread on the Table of the Bread of Presence.

It is possible this bread resembles the Matzoh bread eaten today which is pierced with holes (Leviticus 6:21; Leviticus 24:5-9). If you would like to try making this kind of bread, there is a recipe for making your own matzoh found under the references in the back of the book.

Over and over God instructed the Israelites *"to provide a pleasing aroma to the Lord"* (Exodus 29:18 [ESV]; Genesis 8:21; 25; 41; Leviticus 1:9, 16; Numbers 15:3, 17). Providing a pleasing fragrance was a significant component in their covenant worship. Today scientists know that the *toast-like* aromas or odorants from baking bread are created from only a few of the many chemical compounds found in dough.[xv]

After 40 years of wandering in the desert, Moses died, and Joshua led the Israelites back into the land God had given to Abraham so many years before. God had already instructed Moses on how he was to divide the land between each of the twelve tribes. Today this land would have occupied the area between the borders of modern-day Egypt to the south, Jordan to their east, Syria and Lebanon to the north.

The family of Levi was the only tribe that did not receive land. Why? Because they inherited the priesthood. When priests were presented for consecration, their families were required to bring thick unleavened loaves of bread with olive oil mixed in and thin unleavened bread with olive oil brushed on (Exodus 29:2).

Every year for the First Fruit Offering, grain was taken directly from the threshing floor to the tabernacle (Numbers 15:20). Threshing floors were used to separate the wheat from the chaff by pounding the grains against a large stone slab. Threshing floors were also valued as a good place for worship. King Solomon's temple was built on a threshing floor that King David had purchased from Araunath, who was a Jebusite, not an Israelite (2 Samuel 24:24). A prayer was answered by King David on a threshing floor (1 Chronicles 21:28).

The threshing floor had become a constant metaphor for God's use. The prophet Isaiah had a vision of the people of Israel being crushed on a threshing floor (Isaiah 21:10). The prophet Hosea wrote that Israel would be like chaff in a swirling vortex from the threshing floor if they continued to worship and kiss calf idols (Hosea 13:3). Making bread with or without yeast would have been a task that consumed biblical culture as they experienced God's provision on a personal and national scale with its abundance or scarcity on their threshing floors.

God enlightened the prophets and gave some of them knowledge of a New Covenant which would take place in the future of Israel. Judah was the fourth son of Jacob who received the portion of land around Jerusalem. (Genesis 49; Isaiah 2:2; 42:6; 18:7; Jeremiah 31:31; Daniel 7:14; Luke 22:20; 1 Corinthians 11:25; Hebrews 8:6; 8:8; 8:13; 9:15; 12:24).

> *Behold, the days are coming, declares the Lord, when I will make a new covenant with the house of Israel, and the house of Judah* (Jeremiah 31:31 [ESV]; Hosea 2:23)

The lineage of Jesus can also be traced back through the Biblical book of Ruth. There it describes the meeting and engagement of Ruth and Boaz, which took place around a threshing floor during a harvest season.

Jesus called Himself the Bread of Life (John 6:32-35), and bread was prominent in His ministry. Once, Jesus broke five loaves of bread and used them to feed 5,000 people and had 12 remaining baskets. Was it one basket for each tribe?

Another time Jesus broke seven loaves to feed 4,000 and had seven baskets left. (Mark 8:19-21). Seven, was known for completion and rest. Some people followed Jesus for bread in their bellies, while others were attracted to Jesus for the bread of His fellowship because they had a hunger for His words.

After the last supper Jesus ate with His disciples, He methodically broke the bread and drank the wine with them and asked them to do the same after He was gone. He said to them, *"This is my body which is given for you: this do in remembrance of me"* (Luke 22:19 ESV). Here, Jesus fulfilled the everlasting covenant of bread and established the new covenant, that was to be remembered with bread and wine. (Leviticus 24:8)

After Jesus' crucifixion, resurrection, and ascension; the Apostle Paul wrote:

> *thanks be to God, who always leads us as captives in Christ's triumphal procession and uses us to spread the aroma of the knowledge of him everywhere* (2 Corinthians 2:14 NIV).

When we observe what we call "the Lord's Supper," it is an outward and inward expression of a commitment to choose fellowship with Jesus and eternal life with His heavenly Father.

Today the process of growing, threshing, and grinding grain to make bread is done on an industrial scale and brought to our local stores each morning. Modern men and women have lost the deep personal meaning of sharing in the harvest work, separating the grain from the chaff, grinding and baking the bread before they offer it, eat it, and share it.

Nevertheless, even with all the modern farming technology, the provision of grain is still a critical component of our survival, as populations increase across the earth. We cannot help but be reminded that there is a spiritual connection to bread and life, because without our harvest crops, we are still faced with our own fragility.

Jeremiah wrote that although God led the Israelites out of Egypt like a husband with the pillar of fire by night and the pillar of cloud by day, they still broke their covenant with Him. Then Jeremiah also wrote that someday God would restore Israel, and when He does, the law will be in their minds and in their hearts, and He will be their God and they will be His people (Jeremiah 31:34 paraphrased).

The wise men's gift of frankincense

God required Moses to make holy incense from frankincense along with other fragrant plants for the tabernacle. This incense was only permitted to be prepared and burned by the Levite priests.

Before the birth of Jesus, there was a Levite priest named Zechariah who was married to Elizabeth, and they had no children. Luke wrote that when it was Zechariah's turn to go into the temple and burn incense, he entered the Holy Room, while there were worshipers outside praying. Inside the Holy Room an angel of the Lord appeared to him and stood on the right side of the Altar of Incense. The angel announced to Zechariah that he and his wife Elizabeth would have a son and that they were to name him John (the Baptist). Zechariah was told that John would be filled with the Holy Spirit even before he was born, and that John's life would be dedicated to preparing the people for the coming of the LORD (Jesus).

We know from these passages about Zechariah that the Levite priests were still preparing and burning incense as a requirement of the covenant laws. This was being done in the second Temple at the time of John the Baptist's birth.

The wise men from the east followed a star in the sky to the Israelite city named Bethlehem (which means, *The House of Bread"*). There they gave baby Jesus, Mary, and Joseph gifts of gold, frankincense, and myrrh. The wise men may have even traveled along the Grain Roads where cinnamon, spikenard, other spices, and goods would also come into Jerusalem from a great distance.

The miracle of the wise men, (who were possibly astrologers since they had followed a star) was that they would not have known the Scriptures written by Israel's prophets that predicted the birth of a Great Prophet who would also become King (Matthew 2:1; Genesis 49:10; Numbers 24:17; 2 Samuel 7:26; Isaiah 7:14; 9:6; 11:1; Jeremiah 23:5; 31:15; Hosea 11:1; Micah 5:2). It is surprising that others from outside of Israel were also involved in fulfilling the Scriptures. This is also true in our day.

At the time of Jesus' birth, gold, frankincense, and myrrh were often the gifts that were given to kings. It would have been very unusual for educated and wealthy wise men to enthusiastically leave these kinds of gifts with an Israelite working-class family.

Mary and Joseph were on a journey with the living Son of God, and their heavenly Father provided for their every need. It is feasible that Mary could have used frankincense for diaper burns or scratches that may have become inflamed, or she could have used it for her own personal needs that new mothers often have. To prepare the frankincense, she could have finely ground it on a stone, dropped the powder in olive oil and beeswax, and let it melt on low heat so the oil did not smoke. Then she could have strained it with scraps of linen and allowed it to cool and harden until she had a need for it. Baby Jesus was human and had every need we all have for shelter, food, safety, love, and companionship.

> *But you, O Bethlehem Ephrathah,[4] who are too little to be among the clans of Judah, from you shall come forth for me one who is to be ruler in Israel, whose coming forth is from of old, from ancient days (Micah 5:2 ESV).*

Moses' law required new mothers to come to the temple with their firstborn child for a purification ceremony (Leviticus 12). So at some point after Jesus' birth, Mary and Joseph would have purchased a lamb and a dove (or two doves) for a sin offering for their first-born to consecrate Him to the Lord.

It was on this trip to the temple when they encountered Simeon, a righteous elderly man who was filled with the Spirit and waiting for the consolation of Israel *the Promised One* (Genesis 12:1-3). Simeon declared that baby Jesus was "*a light for revelation of the Gentiles, and for glory to your people Israel"* (Luke 2:32 ESV). While they were still at the temple, Joseph and Mary also met Anna, a prophet, who never left the temple. When she saw baby Jesus, she thanked God and

---

[4] *Ephrathah*, another name for fruitful.

spoke about Him as the *"redemption of Jerusalem"* (Luke 2:38).

Simeon was not described as a priest or prophet but as a righteous old man. So from his example we know that others in Israel also had the gift of prophecy. Anna is called a prophet but we never read about an official anointing of women designated to serve as a prophetess, and yet she is acknowledged as one. This reminds us of a powerful truth: God has not left mankind alone; His plan has always included a way for us to return to Him and to know and acknowledge His work.

Other prophecies about Christ *"the Anointed One"* can also be found in: Genesis 3:15; Deuteronomy 18:15; Isaiah 11:12; 53:5; Haggai 2:6-9; Daniel 9:24-27; Psalm 16:7-11; 22; 34:20; 110:1-7; Samuel 7:14; Zechariah 9:9; 10:12, and there are many more. Jesus' coming was not hidden from His people.

Jesus was conceived by the Holy Spirit and given birth to by the virgin Mary, making Him all God and Son of Man. He experienced emotions of fear, anger, sorrow, loneliness, and temptation; but He did not react to any of this by sinning. Jesus also experienced hunger and pain, but He had a relationship with His heavenly Father that sustained Him far beyond what we can only imagine. Mary could have also treasured away some of her tears of frankincense to give as an offering to the temple in Jerusalem upon her arrival.

> *Behold the virgin shall conceive and bear a son, and shall call his name Immanuel* (Isaiah 7:14 ESV). [5]

Every year in the month of December, we are reminded of these events in a special way when we smell the fragrances that so many of us associate with the Christmas story. In some parts of the world frankincense and myrrh are still used

---

[5] Immanuel means, God with us.

to remind people of the birth of Jesus with gifts of the Wise Men. In the west the fragrances of Douglas firs, Canadian firs, White pines, oranges, cloves, cinnamon, and other aromas are associated with Christmas, which depends on your family's traditions.

When I smell pine, I remember my family's Christmas tree with a manger scene where I spent hours playing with the lights and the characters in the Christmas story. The aroma of pine has always been heavenly for me, as my thoughts go to what I know about heaven, its messengers, and its message from above. Some of my other memories include the prickle from the pine needles on my hands and the sticky fragrant sap on the bark I encountered when I watered the tree.

Very seldom is fragrance used intentionally with learning, even though it is one of the most powerful senses for memory our Creator implanted in us.

$$\approx A\Omega \approx$$

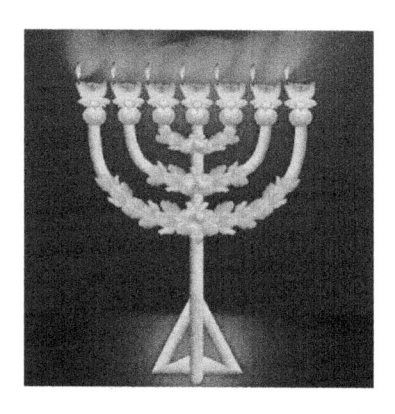

Chapter 3

Olive Oil and Wine for the Bridegroom

Make a fragrant offering of oil and wine

Display olive oil in glass, fresh olives, olive wood, or a potted olive tree. Arrange bunches of black or red grapes. Display new or old grape juice in a glass or arrange grape leaves and vines in a wreath.

Plant name for oil: Olive oil, or *Olea europaea subsp. Cerasiformis (NT)* is near threatened. The Greek writer Homer called olive oil "liquid gold," and the Greek doctor Hippocrates called it "the great healer."[xvi]

Olive tree family: Oleaceae which includes the lilac, jasmine, forsythia, and ash.[xvii]

Plant name for wine: Indigenous grape vines in Israel were abandoned under Muslim occupation in 636 AD. Since the late 1800s, Israel has grown and produced Kosher-Cabernet Sauvignon, and *Vitis vinifera,* along with some others.

Grape plant family: Vitaceae, from the genus Vitis.

Oil and wine extraction/characteristics: Olive oil is a heavy oil with a yellowish-green color that is retrieved from the pulp of the fruit rather than the seed. This oil is thick and not always the first choice for massage because of its density it will not glide over the skin easily. It is not ideal for cooking at high temperatures because it smokes, which we now know can be toxic for people. It is best served raw on salads and vegetables. Olive oil contains large amounts of antioxidants and have anti-inflammatory properties. Vegetable oils are lipids, composed of fatty acids that are a vital source of energy and are used for building and maintaining the cells in our body. When olive oil is cold pressed without heat it maintains its vital nutrients.

Grape juice was extracted by stomping the grapes. Original storage and aging of wine was in wineskins or animal hides from goat or sheep. Both oil and wine were extracted in vats or large flat stone containers with a spout.

Aroma and taste of olive oil: Olive oil has a green, nutty smell and taste. When fresh olive oil is swallowed by itself, the antioxidants will briefly burn or bite the soft tissue in the back of the throat. Some people may find this trait of fresh olive oil unpleasant.

Aroma of wine: The aroma of Cabernet Sauvignon is described to smell like violets, blackcurrant, cedar, and spice when grown today in Bordeaux. However, the aroma and flavor of wine will depend on many conditions, including what type of wood in which the wine is aged in. The aroma and taste of wine aged in wineskins would have tasted and smelled flat and gamey compared to today's wine. When grape juice is aged in wineskins the flavor and aroma are not as rewarding because the complex chemicals in the wood which cause aromatic changes in the wine that benefit its flavor.

Biblical references for olive oil

- The recipe for the holy anointing oil used olive oil as the base ingredient (Exodus 30:24).
- Olive oil was used to burn the lamps on the lampstand (Leviticus 24:2; 2 Chronicles 4:7).
- Oil was also used for the offering of unleavened bread and was placed on the Table of the Bread of Presence in the temple (Exodus 29:2).
- In addition, olive oil was also required to be offered with the first sacrificial lamb at dawn (Exodus 29:40).
- Strong wine (undiluted) and olive oil were both required as an offering or tithe (giving the Lord ten percent of their profits) so the temple so the priests could carry out their duties for the drink offering along with the burnt offering required each morning (Numbers 28:7).
- Anointing someone's head with oil was a sign of hospitality or as a way to acknowledge and elevate their social status (Luke 7:46).
- David said God anointed his head with oil and his cup overflowed (Psalm 23:5). God's love is compared to an olive tree (Psalms 52:8). Possibly because the olive tree is abundant in the fruit that could be understood as anointing.
- Cherubim, palm trees and open flowers were carved into the olive wood temple doors (1 Kings 6:31).
- Zechariah the priest had a vision of the gold lampstand and olive trees (Zechariah 4:1-14).
- Virgin olive oil was most likely the oil used by the disciples to anoint the sick as part of the prayer for healing (James 5:14).

Biblical references for wine

- Abraham and the Great High Priest Melchizedek shared wine and bread together (Genesis 14:18).
- A prophetic verse written about Christ in Genesis, *"he will wash his garments in wine, and his robes in the blood of grapes"* (Genesis 49:11 NIV).
- The Levites were instructed not to drink wine while serving in the tabernacle (Leviticus 10:8).
- The Israelites tithed wine and olive oil (Deuteronomy 18:4).
- The vow of the Nazarite for a man or woman included not drinking wine (Numbers 6:1-4; Judges 13:13; Jeremiah 35:8).
- King David wrote about wine mixed with spices (Psalms 75:8). This could have been similar to what the English drink for the Christmas holidays (spiced wine) which includes cinnamon, nutmeg, and orange skins.
- No priest was to drink wine before entering the inner court (Ezekiel 44:21).
- The prophet Daniel abstained from wine (Daniel 10:3).

Essence of Day

- The Priest Zechariah was instructed by an angel of the Lord not to give wine to his son John the Baptist (Luke 1:15).
- Jesus' first miracle at a wedding in Cana, was turning water into wine (John 2:3-10).
- Wine represents the blood of Christ, while the bread represents His body (1Corinthians 10:16).

Historical application of olive oil and wine

Olive oil was essential for the ancient people who lived around the Mediterranean. There would have been olive-oil tasters just like there are wine tasters today. Each region around the Mediterranean has its own unique flavor of oil. The process of growing olive trees and making olive oil may have begun as early as 2400 BC[xviii] (Goodfellow).

Olive oil is extremely nutritious. It is also soothing to dry, cracked or crepe skin, and is good for abrasions and wounds. It can even be used to condition the scalp and hair. Not all vegetable oils are suitable for use on the scalp and hair. It was used as fuel for the ancients' lamps, an important part of nutrition in their diet, and an element of self-care.

The hot climate in the Middle East is drying to the skin. Using soap with clean water carried by hand would have been a limited option. The prophet Jeremiah mentioned that the use of soap and cleansing powder was not able to wash away people's guilt (Jeramiah 2:22). Soap was made with lye, derived from hardwood ash and a fat such as olive oil.

As you can clearly see, olive oil permeated the way of life 2,000 years ago in the lands described in the Bible. It was cultivated, processed, and traded as a vital part of their economy then, and the same is still being done today in many countries like Spain, Italy, Greece, and in whole geographic areas like the Middle East.

Oil became synonymous with several things:

- The flame or light on the Lampstand; providing light to those in spiritual darkness; and the anointing of the Spirit with joy (Isaiah 61:3).
- To anoint one's body with oil appears to be a way for a person to make themselves presentable to others for a special occasion (Ruth 3:3; Micah 6:15).
- To anoint the head of a visitor to your home appears to have been intended to give them a place of honor, or simply to make them feel extra welcome (Luke:7:46).
- James and the twelve disciples used oil when they laid their hands on the sick and prayed (Mark 6:13; James 5:14).
- God instantaneously anoints our soul (with the fruit of the Spirit) when we come to realize we are His children and ask Him to make us His own.

Historical application of wine: diluted with water (50%—50%) made water safe enough to ingest before modern water purification became common. Wine, or vinegar and oil, were also used as a base liquid for macerating (soaking) herbs for medicine. Oil and wine were frequently used to clean a wound which would have been soothing and disinfecting (Luke 10:34).

Grape plants are woody perennial vines which require full sun exposure to produce fruit. Flowers and fruit grow out from new shoots off of the main vines. Annual pruning is essential for growing fruit. In general, vineyards require a lot of labor and time to keep the plants healthy and disease free. Israel was referred to as a vineyard (Isaiah 5:1-7). Jesus used the properties of the grape plant to illustrate what kind of relationship we need to keep with Him so we may also bear the fruit of the Spirit.

> *If you remain in me, and I in you, you will bear much fruit; apart from me you can do nothing* (John 15:5 NIV).

Oil for the seven lamps on the lampstand

God gave Moses the ten commandment laws and many other supporting laws for everyday life, so the Israelites would know how to live with each other and with Himself (Deuteronomy 5:7-22). God also provided Moses with a pattern to build a tabernacle so He could dwell inside the camp with the Israelites (Exodus 25:8-9). The design for the tabernacle included six altars which had special requirements including the use of fragrant plants, oils, and incense. Olive oil was required for use in the holy anointing oil for consecrating the tabernacle and the priests, as well as for fuel in the lampstand. It was also required for use with the bread and burnt offerings.

The outside of the tabernacle was a tent made from woven goat hair. It had two main rooms divided by curtains. The first room was rectangularly shaped and was called the "Holy Room." Inside the Holy Room there were three articles for worship. The solid gold lampstand sat on the left-hand side of the tabernacle and it weighed Seventy-five pounds, (33 Kilo/one talent). It stood opposite the Table of the Bread of Presence with its lamps facing forward and oblique, directing its light toward the Altar of Incense. The Altar of Incense sat in front of the veil (or shielding curtain) which was just outside of the Most Holy Room. The Most Holy Room was a very sacred forbidden space that was only entered one time a year by the great high priest for the forgiveness of sin. God's presence filled this space which was in the shape of a square. Inside of the Most Holy Room was the Ark of the Covenant also called the "Mercy Seat."

The lampstand is described in great detail in Exodus 25:31. It was solid gold and weighed 75 pounds (33 kilos or one talent). It had a main shaft in the center which held the middle lamp and six ornate stems to the sides which held three more lamps. Each lamp had a solid gold saucer where the lamps would sit. The design of the lampstand was modeled after the almond trees, leaves and fruit.

Aaron the priest entered the tabernacle at dusk after he had washed in the basin. He would first light the Altar of Incense, and then he would light each of the seven lamps, all of which were to be kept burning all night. At twilight Aaron would return to first light the incense and, then snuff out each of the lamps. In preparation for that evening he would trim the wicks, clean, and refill each gold lamp with oil so it would be ready to relight again at dusk. This was to be repeated day after day and evening after evening throughout the future generations as an everlasting covenant. God had planned every detail for covenant worship in the tabernacle, including the way that each of the altars was to be used. The altar of incense held a prominent position.

For approximately 2,500 years, excluding the years the Israelites spent in exile, they had tried but failed to keep the whole covenant law. God knew the law was going to be too hard for the people to follow in its entirety, but this was a way for God to not only show Israel their sin, but also to reveal His bigger plan. He showed them all of this within the pattern, function and actions of the priests within the tabernacle. Covenant worship gave Israel hope and reminded them and their future generations that God was still with them.

God also gave Moses laws for everyday living, rules to keep order and to help resolve disputes. These laws are found in the first five books of the Old Testament, called the "Torah." God wanted His people to know there was a better way for them to live their days on the earth, a way that would ultimately lead them to eternal life. They understood there was a requirement for righteousness they would have found impossible to fully obtain, if it was not for God who is compassionate and merciful (Exodus 34:6-7; Romans 8:4).

The ten bridesmaids and the Bridegroom

Jesus told a parable about ten virgins who were invited to a wedding festival. Five of them carried extra olive oil for their lamps, but five of the them failed to prepare themselves with extra oil in case the bridegroom arrived late. When Jesus told this story of the ten bridesmaids, he used it to preview his return to the earth. Each person would need to be prepared, but even with a warning some would still fail to be ready.

Essence of Day

Bridesmaids in ancient Israel may have carried a small vial of extra oil on the end of a strap for the purpose of refilling their lamps. During Jesus' time, oil lamps were small, terracotta, circular, and flat, not much bigger than the palm of a hand. There was a hole in the middle where the lamp was filled. The lamp had a spout from which the wick protruded for the flame to burn. There was often a small, stubby handle one could use to help support the lamp in their hand with a thumb and finger. The lamp could only burn for a few hours before it would need refilling.

There were other plants also cultivated for oil in Israel, such as nut oil from the almond, flax seed oil and grapeseed oil, but it was olive oil from the fruit that remained central for their diet, culture, personal use, and for the worship of Yahweh.

The Gospels of Matthew, Mark, Luke and John all agree that Jesus referred to Himself as a Bridegroom. Even Jesus' first miracle was performed at a wedding in Cana, after the bridegroom had run out of wine for his guests (John 2:1-12). Jesus had the servants (who knew exactly from where the wine had come) gather water into the empty vats. He turned that water into wine that was even better tasting than what had already been served! When the wedding planner tasted the wine, he was surprised and remarked, how the host had kept the good wine until the last (John 2:10). Two important messages in this story are that the servants knows and shares in the father's work, and for those who wait, the best is reserved for last.

Why did Jesus perform His first miracle at a wedding? Perhaps he wanted to make a point:

> *For this reason, a man will leave his father and mother and be united to his wife, and the two will become one flesh. This is a profound mystery—but I am talking about Christ and the church* (Ephesians 5:31-32 NIV). Isaiah 62:5; Hosea 2:19.

The evening before Jesus' death He led the disciples to the Mount of Olives, where they passed over the Kidron valley. The Kidron was known for its fast-moving water in the rainy season. This valley separated the high point of Jerusalem from the Mount of Olives and eventually emptied into the Dead Sea. On this evening the air around the Kidron valley may still have lingered with the fragrant smoke from hundreds or even thousands of chosen lambs that had been sacrificed and grilled with natural hardwood charcoal briquets for Passover. Jesus would have completely understood why His heavenly Father had established the everlasting covenant law of sacrifice, as He and the disciples walked through the valley of the shadow of death, in order to arrive at the Mount of Olives. Hundreds of years before Jesus birth the prophet Zechariah received advance notice and wrote,

> *One day the Lord will return with all the holy ones with Him and will stand on the Mount of Olives after which a great earthquake will take place that will split the ground from the east to west with the mountain moving north and south. On this day there will be no separation of day and night; instead it will remain light as the Lord reigns* (Zechariah 14:4-9 paraphrased).

When I use olive oil, I imagine the light from Creation that pierced the emptiness and separated light from darkness like oil completely separates from water. Then I remember the last night Jesus labored in prayer on the Mount of Olives, and held fast to God's covenant promise, to provide a way to separate our sin and remove our transgressions far away for us. (Psalm 103:12)

$$\approx A\Omega \approx$$

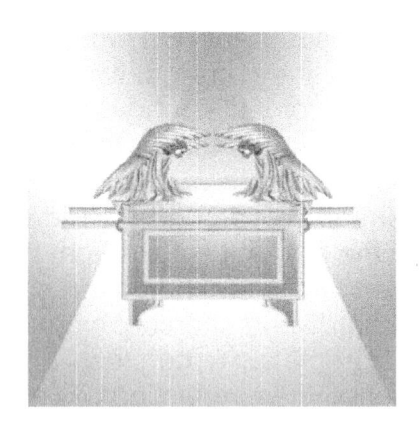

Chapter 4:

Acacia Wood for the Day of Atonement

The fragrant offering of acacia

You can make a crown of thorns with acacia wood or hawthorn if you are in North America. Feel free to make an acacia flower arrangement if you have this plant with its yellow or pink blossoms.

Plant name for acacia: *Acacia seyal.* Family: Mimosa. Acacia wood was a common hardwood in the Bible lands. The country of origin is Senegal in Africa, but there are now over 400 species found around the world. The name for acacia wood in Hebrew is *"'shittah' or 'shittim'"* (plural) meaning *"to pierce"* no doubt because of its thorns.[6]

Oil extraction/characteristics: The wood is not harvested for its aroma or essential oil, but rather some varieties are harvested for their roots and flowers. The tree wood is known for its durability and density as a hardwood, but it has large

---
[6] Strong's Number: 07850 Original Word: ttX. Word Origin: root meaning (to pierce). Transliterated Word: *Shotet.* Definition: Scourge.

woody thorns. Some types of acacia also produce a gum resin used as a food additive or as a syrup or thickener to help make a sweet drink easier to swallow.

Aroma: Some varieties of acacia have aromatic yellow flowers that are used for making perfume. The wood is not used for its aromatics.

Biblical references for acacia wood

- When Moses went up to Mount Sinai, he took an ark (chest) he had made out of acacia wood that he would use to house the stone tablets (Deuteronomy 10:3).
- Moses was also instructed by God to use acacia wood in the construction of certain parts of the tabernacle (Exodus 36:36).
- The Ark of the Covenant was made from acacia and covered with gold (Exodus 37).
- The Ark of the Covenant was placed in the Most Holy Room and was only approached one time a year.
- Four of the six altars were made from acacia wood.
- Isaiah wrote that Israel should not fear, because God would not forsake them, in fact, God would provide acacia, myrtle, olive and cypress trees (Isaiah 41:19).
- What about the thorns? We're told that Jesus was *"pierced for our transgressions"* (Isaiah 53:5 NIV). In line with this, there was also the strange occurrence when the Roman soldiers fashioned a crown of thorns and pushed it into his head.

Historical application of acacia wood

Acacia is a common type of hardwood in the Middle East, used often because of its durability. Splints, canes, staffs, and stretchers could have been made from this wood, as well as carts, axles, wheels and tent poles.

Acacia seyal or Acacia Senegal are most likely the type of wood used in the tabernacle. There are over a hundred varieties of this species, which is related to the mimosa.[xix] Acacia wood is not harvested for its fragrant wood, although mimosa blossoms are used to make an exotic absolute, which is a process used for capturing the fragrance of flowers to make perfume. *Acacia farnesiana* or Cassie is a variety of mimosa that is processed for its flowers. Its fragrance is obtained by using solvent extraction with hexane on the flowers. It is a slow, expensive process that goes through a number of steps to obtain a fragrant oily substance called "concrete." Impurities are removed from the concrete and the final absolute or fragrant liquid is retrieved.

This slow process can be used for many different kinds of flowers petals, including roses. The fragrance of this particular mimosa flower is extremely warm, powdery, herbaceous, and floral with a violet top note. It has a tenacious cinnamic-balsamic dry out.[xx] The *dry out* or *dry down* is the end note, or the last fragrance your nose is able to detect. Quite often the first fragrance you detect is a top note that changes as your olfactory receptors adjust to the whole chemical compound and the notes blend or dry down.

Local bees are attracted to the mimosa's fragrant, brightly colored flowers, and their honey also takes on its special, beneficial chemical characteristics and fragrance. Making the point that aromatic plant chemicals also enter our bodies through our stomach.

Acacia seyal is a very dense hardwood similar to the Osage orange or hedge apple found in North America. *Acacia seyal* and *Acacia senegal* also exudes a gum resin called gum Arabic. The resin, bark, and roots of the acacia can all be used to retrieve the useful gum. This may have been the "gum resin" used in the holy incense, but there were also other plants in the area that produced gum resin's (Exodus 30:34 NIV).

In ancient Egypt acacia gum resin was used as an adhesive to glue layers of linen together for making mummies. Acacia is still harvested there today for flavoring food, soft drinks, and candy, and it even has some nutritional value.[xxi] This hardwood had many uses for the Israelites, but its large woody thorns also reminded them (and us) of the curse of thorns. Acacia wood used for the tabernacle altars may have also been important because of its spiritual significance related to the curse of thorns. The Genesis account of original sin stated that the earth was also impacted negatively by Adam's sin, and along with us it is also suffering its effects.

The Tabernacle and the Ark of the Covenant

The Lord spoke to Moses saying, *"Let them make a sanctuary; that I may dwell in their midst"* (Exodus 25:8 ESV). God provided every detail of the tabernacle for Moses to use in its construction. It was to be a tent, that could be taken down and put back up as the Israelites wandered in the desert for 40 years. Acacia wood poles were used to hold up the tent.

God required Moses to make four of the six altars used for worship in the tabernacle out of acacia wood. Three of these altars were used inside the tabernacle and were made from acacia wood and covered with gold. The Ark of the Covenant was considered the most holy altar and it was placed inside the Most Holy Room. The ark was adorned with gold cherubim on its lid, also called the mercy seat. These cherubim were kneeling at both ends with their wings touching over the exact middle of the ark (Exodus 25:17-22).

As we read earlier, the Ark of the Covenant was only approached by the high priest once a year, on the Day of Atonement. Inside the Ark were the ten-commandment stone tablets God gave to Moses on Mount Sinai. According to an author of the Talmud, written in Aramaic during Israel's Babylonian captivity, the Ark of the Covenant could have also contained the broken tablets (Moses had broken when he found the people sinning by worshiping the golden calf). [7]

---

[7] Sefaria, Inc. *The William Davidson Talmud*, bava batra 14b, https://www.sefaria.org/Bava_Batra.14b?lang=bi. [Accessed 05-14-2020]

The ark also contained a pot of manna from the desert, along with Aaron's staff (Moses brother) which had bloomed and sprouted almond buds, blooms, and ripe almonds at a critical time in their history (Exodus 16:33-34; Numbers 17:8-10).

When all the requirements God gave Moses for the tabernacle were met including the required animal sacrifices, the burning of the holy incense and the consecration with the holy anointing oil, the Lord rested on the tabernacle and spoke to Moses face to face, like a man speaks to his friend (Exodus 33:11).

After the construction of King Solomon's temple, there were two more cherubim added to the temple. They were carved from olive wood and covered with gold. These cherubim also stood in the Most Holy Room of the temple and had wings which extended across the width of the room, almost touching the walls at one end and each other at the center. They stood over the Ark of the Covenant with it's two other cherubim.

All these Cherubim symbolized the entry or gateway back to our Creator God as they kneeled and stood at attention over the law inside Ark of the Covenant. This altar was a powerful symbol of the everlasting covenant God had made with Israel. The ornamentations in the tabernacle were important to aid the Israelites in understanding God's Holiness. Later, the prophet Jeremiah wrote that Israel had become unfaithful and as a result the Ark of the Covenant would be forgotten:

> *It shall not come to mind or be remembered or missed; it shall not be made again* (Jeremiah 3:16 ESV).

So what was the purpose of the Ark of the Covenant? God was and has always been more concerned with the unseen condition of our innermost being, which results in actions that either befit or defile us, much more than He has been concerned with our performance in worship of Him (Mark 7:21-23). Once we acknowledge, confess and repent from our fallen condition, He will begin to transform, heal, and change us from deep within.

This is similar to the influence of a plant fragrance. At times, fragrance may affect us so deeply that we cannot understand it in a logical way. But even then, there is observable evidence that can be seen in our countenance, and in our choices going forward. These fragrances also effects change for the better, not only in our lives but in our environment. Acacia wood with its round soft, delicate, hair-like, pink or yellow halo of aromatic blossoms on its branch of thorns can also be displayed to create a fragrant memory of Jesus' crucifixion as He was pierced for the forgiveness of our sin.

Linen and the Day of Atonement

Another important plant product for worship of Yahweh is linen. Flax or *Linum usitatissimum* is from the family of plants called Linaceae. It is one of the oldest known cultivated plants that grow in and around the Mediterranean. Flax has medicinal properties of its own and its oil is commonly used for constipation, inflammation, and the reduction of cholesterol levels. The seeds and the oil from food grade flax can also be consumed.

Flax stems contain cellulose fibers that have traditionally been dried, spun, and woven on looms into linen, a skill which dates back to the fifth millennium BC. Linen was tithed for the construction of the tabernacle, specifically for the curtains which served as inside walls of the tabernacle. Moses wrote that the Lord moved the hearts of every skillful woman who spun linen or goat hair with her hands, and that they gave blue, purple, or scarlet yarn for the construction of the temple (Exodus 35:25-26).

Linen was also used for the priestly garments. It included the cloth for the ephod which was a decorative outer garment or vestment with twelve different gemstones in three rows of four.

The ephod was worn on the priest's chest on top of another linen garment.

Anointing oil and linen were used together on the day of Yom Kippur or the "Day of Atonement." Most Rabbis believe Yom Kippur first occurred after Moses had been on Mount Sinai for 40 days when he had received the first set of ten-commandment stone tablets from God. On his return to camp he discovered the Israelites had built, and were worshiping, a golden calf. What made it worse is that Aaron his own brother was leading the blasphemy. Moses broke the tablets and destroyed the idol. After he burned it, he ground it down, and made the Israelites drink the gold dust and ash (Exodus 32:20).

When God threatened to destroy the Israelites, Moses fasted, prayed and pleaded for over another 40 days, and asked for God to forgive Aaron and the Israelites for their sin of idolatry. The first commandment on tablets stated, *"You shall have no other gods before me"* (Exodus 20:3 ESV).

On the Day of Atonement, the Israelites were required to sacrifice a red bull and burn parts of it outside the walls of Jerusalem. Anything outside of Jerusalem was considered unclean but the place where the red bull was burned was consider clean and sacred.

On this Holy Day the high priest performed the required sacrifices and then prepared himself to enter the Most Holy Room. He did not wear the ephod but first bathed in the temple area and then donned the sacred linen garment which included a linen turban and a linen sash around his waist (Exodus 16). It appears this garment was used again and again and was even passed down to Aaron's sons. This garment was not to leave the tabernacle. After the anointing was complete, the priest would remove the garment, bathe again, and put his own clothing back on, all done in the temple area (Leviticus 16:23).

Today the Jews still celebrate the Day of Atonement as their most important annual holy day. The only other holy day of similar importance is the weekly Sabbath Day, because it had been written into the Ten Commandment stones as the fourth commandment.

Did God establish any of the religious rituals for Israel because of their need for some kind of beatification or cleansing, since they had just come out of Egypt's culture of idol worship? Possibly, but Covenant worship at its core bound Israel to God's promises with exercises requiring their obedience, all as a pattern and a copy for things that were still to come.

The cross and the crown of thorns

Although the Bible does not tell us what wood was used for the cross Jesus was crucified on, it is an interesting thought that the cross could have been cut out of acacia wood. The Roman guards fashioned thorns into a crown for Jesus which may have been nearby as leftovers from hewing the hardwood crosses.

Jesus was pierced for our sins, died, and rose from the grave, providing a way to eradicate sin and death once and for all. When the Romans lifted Jesus up on the cross and placed a crown of thorns on His head, their intent was to make fun of Him as King of the Jews.

According to Roman law, to claim you were a king was punishable by death. For the Israelites, the thorns signified the curse of sin and death, as it had been recorded in the book of Genesis. Did God have all this in mind when He instructed Moses in every last detail for the tabernacle, including the type of wood used for the altars?

> *They serve at the sanctuary that is a copy and shadow of what is in heaven* (Hebrews 8:5 NIV).

The next time I have the opportunity to inhale the warm, powdery, herbaceous, violet top note of the soft pink mimosa flowers, I will look for its thorns, and will remember the pain I have also caused by my sin. I will recall the curse of sin and how God still chose to provide for me when His One and Only Son was scourged, wore the crown of thorns, was pierced on the cross for my sins, died, and was placed in the tomb.

The story didn't end there. Jesus rose from the dead, walked with His followers, and then ascended into the heavens. If we accept His salvation with a confession of faith, we too will be resurrected and will once again walk with God.

$$\approx A\Omega \approx$$

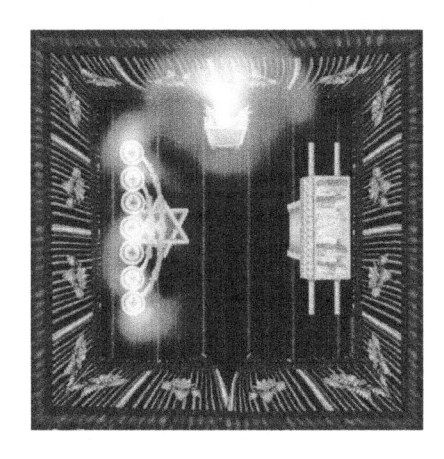

Chapter 5

Myrrh, Consecration, and The Altar of Burnt Offering

Make a fragrant offering of myrrh

"*Stacte*" is used in some translations of the Bible, which translates to a sweet resin or myrrh. You can present fresh myrrh resin, diluted myrrh essential oil, or provide a fragrant myrrh candle or soap.

Plant name: *Commiphora myrrha*. Family: Burseraceae. From the Mediterranean, western Asia, Tunisia, France, Corsica, Spain, Morocco and Italy.[xxii] The root wood of myrrh means "bitter."

Oil extraction/characteristics: Today myrrh resin is ground into a powder and steam distilled to produce essential oil. The holy anointing oil was most likely macerated or prepared like a balm which would have been heated and the impurities strained out. The essential oil ranges from yellow to orange in color. The orifice reducing cap on my bottle of myrrh oxidizes and sticks, which makes it hard to open even when it is fresh and safe to use. This is typical for myrrh but not for other oils, when they oxidize, they are actually no longer safe to use.

Aroma: Myrrh has a sharp, woody, balsamic, alcohol, and a medicinal-like top note (like described by Septimus Piesse the perfumer from France who notes to describe fragrances).

Emotional benefits: Myrrh instills a deep sense of calm and tranquility in the mind.[xxiii] This may not be true for everyone, especially if the medicinal top note triggers a fear of a medical office, or they associate the smell with another negative experience.

Biblical references for myrrh

- Joseph's brothers sold him into slavery to a passing caravan loaded with spice, balm, and myrrh. Afterwards Jacob sent his sons back to Egypt with gifts, including myrrh (Genesis 43:11).
- Olive oil and myrrh were the base ingredients in the holy anointing oil. This compound was used for the consecration of the altars, the tabernacle and later the temples and was used to anoint the priests (Leviticus 8:10-30).
- The book of Esther recorded that myrrh was also used for Esther's beauty preparations (Esther 1:12). Myrrh was for the preservation of health and beauty.
- Myrrh was mentioned as a sachet which is a cloth bag containing myrrh that could have been worn (Song of Solomon 1:13).
- The wise men gave myrrh to baby Jesus after His birth.
- Myrrh and or gall were offered to Jesus on the cross by the Roman guards, as a medicinal drink.
- Nicodemus provided a mixture with myrrh when they laid Jesus in the new tomb to be used for burial spices (Matthew 27:66).
- We have become vessels of God and are anointed by the Spirit for His good work (1 John 2:20; 2:27).
- Christos (Christ) is Jesus' Greek title, meaning "the Anointed One."

Historical application of myrrh

Some of the benefits for myrrh are its anti-inflammatory, antimicrobial, antiseptic, astringent, and cicatrisant (helps regenerate cells). It can also be used as a fungicidal, as well as for bedsores and wounds.[xxiv] Use of myrrh is over 4000 years old in Egypt.[xxv]

Myrrh is a shrub with thorns. It produces a sap that seeps through the bark and then hardens. The bark can be cut to revive or increase the flow of resin. The sap dries into a dark reddish-brown resin that falls to the ground and is collected.

Today, ground resin is steam distilled to retrieve the essential oil, but in ancient times they would have also ground myrrh resin and heated or macerated it in olive oil, until the aroma and plant chemicals were released. Myrrh's effect on our moods or emotion is similar to that of frankincense. Some have reported that it helps one discover inner stillness and peace, freeing us from restlessness so we can focus on the spiritual or unseen part of our lives. Myrrh and frankincense are not the only plants that people report will calm their mood. There are many other plants that are reported to do the same thing, including lavender, cedarwood, ylang ylang and many more.

You might be asking yourself, how is it that plants can affect our mood and improve our awareness of spiritual things? Plants were created to interact with their environment by releasing substances or chemicals that we perceive as a fragrance. These are called plant volatiles. These volatiles or aromas were created to sedate or repulse creatures that might like to eat the plant. Likewise, these same plant volatiles may attract or stimulate other insects that are needed for its pollination. Some plants also have antifungal and antibacterial properties to keep fungus and bacteria from growing on the plants and harming them. In some cases, plants have healing or anti-inflammatory agents called antitranspirants which include acetylsalicylic acid, or salicin a compound used to make aspirin[xxvi].

The reason plants produce analgesic compounds is to numb or deaden an insect, to deter it from harming the plant. Humans also have olfactory receptors for these plant chemicals, and we can be affected by them at some level. For example, lavender and black pepper are useful for the treatment of pain, because they are analgesic. Some aromatherapists, who use fragrant oils on the skin do not think it is necessary to prefer or enjoy a fragrance in order for it to be effective for helping pain. However, most of us would agree that people need to feel comfortable with a fragrance in order to get relief from anxiety or a mood disorder. If a negative association with a plant develops, such as pain from thorns or a rash from an allergic reaction, one will learn to avoid that plant. This would encourage people to investigate other plants for their needs instead. Just like insects, humans are also affected by fragrant chemicals with their various positive or negative associations.

The exception is that humans also develop a hedonistic reaction to fragrances. We learn to enjoy the scent of plants that we like, for example the smell of our favorite meal or the aroma of an apple pie cooking.

The reverse is also true. If we are exposed over and over to the same enjoyable scent in connection with a negative situation, we may learn to dislike that scent even if we used to enjoy it. Another interesting example is when we go to the doctor's office where we might smell isopropyl alcohol along with other strong-smelling cleaning agents. When our visits are repeated too many times because of pain or an illness, we may become conditioned to react cautiously when entering a new room with that same odor.

When we have learned to associate a negative experience with a fragrance and encounter that fragrance again in the future, it is likely to cause anxiety or even fear. Some negative reactions to fragrance might be so intense they even increase our heart rate and blood pressure. The opposite can also be true, when positive reactions to a fragrance might calm us, reducing our heart rate and blood pressure.

Fragrances are connected to our health in some other surprising ways. There have been studies that suggest they improve our immune system. Our immune system is complex, but God gave us many instinctive ways to build it up and keep it strong.

The loss of smell or *anosmia* is one of the first signs of specific diseases. These include Alzheimer's, Huntington's, Paget's, Parkinson's, and Schizophrenia. More recently, we have learned that it is one of the first symptoms of COVID-19.

One can also experience an olfactory hallucination which is called "phantosmia." This can be a sign of a brain tumor, sinus inflammation, a seizure or Parkinson's disease. If you are experiencing this you should definitely seek medical attention. This is one of the most interesting of all the olfactory disorders, because it demonstrates how our sense of smell is so interwoven into our brain. Our olfactory sense can also have an intense reaction related to a memory, a response that seems to come out of nothing.

Our Creator designed us to live and work within the Garden of Eden, which in return gave up her fragrances and fruits to provide for us. Has fragrance been used to alleviate emotional pain and suffering ever since our separation from the garden? I believe the fascination with fragrances have been with us from the very beginning. Basil, bergamot (type of orange), cedarwood, geranium, lavender, patchouli, rose, and ylang ylang are a few other plants provided by God to help alleviate some of our stresses and anxieties.

We may find it difficult to imagine a world free from emotional pain, hunger, physical pain, mental illness, anxiety, fear, disease, abuse and ultimately separation by death. But such a world is indeed coming. Israel's prophets, priests, and kings recorded that a new day is coming when we will live free from all of these afflictions.

> *He will wipe away every tear from their eyes, and death shall be no more, neither shall there be morning, or crying, nor pain anymore,* (Rev 21:4 ESV).

The stench of death will no longer exist, because all that was, will have passed away.

Myrrh in the Holy Anointing Oil

We know from Israel's history that the Levites were appointed as priests to serve in the temple. Some of these priests were filled with the Spirit and in addition were also prophets. So what is the definition of a prophet? Let's look at the life of Moses. Moses had a relationship with God. He followed God's directions, and he remained faithful in his service and intercession of Israel. Scripture made it clear even Moses was not perfect when he errored in anger, it disqualified him from entering the promise land.

The prophet Moses had his first encounter with God on Mount Sinai, when God appeared to him in a burning bush. The Israelites came to understand from their experiences with Moses that there was a deep connection between flames and the Spirit. Mount Sinai had fire on it when the Israelites approached it. God led the Israelites in the desert with a pillar of fire. The lampstand in the tabernacle used oil to make a flame. The use of oil and anointing in the church appears to have lost cultural spiritual and social meaning for us, but for the Israelites oil seems to be a catalyst for God's presence.

The first time we discover anointing in the Bible is in the book of Genesis, when Jacob anointed a pillar after God appeared to him in a dream and promised to bless all the families of the earth through his family (Genesis 28). We will not read about anointing again until God instructed Moses to anoint the altars and articles in the tabernacle, and to anointed Aaron to perform the duties of the high priest (Exodus 40:9-13).

The anointing God established with Moses for the tabernacle and the priests appears to be an outward sign to confirm an increase in spiritual status. Priests were consecrated by sprinkling their garments with the sacrificial blood mixed with anointing oil and by pouring the anointing oil on their head (Exodus 29:21).

When Moses complained to the Lord that the people of Israel were too much for him to handle, the Lord instructed him to choose 70 worthy men, *"And say to the people 'Consecrate yourselves for tomorrow"* (Numbers 11:18 ESV). Then after Moses appointed these men, the Spirit of the Lord rested on the elders and they prophesied and the Holy Spirit spoke through them.

The important thing to note here is that these 70 men had a choice to consecrate themselves before the Lord. We are not told whether or not they consecrated themselves with blood or oil. I imagine they did at least use oil as an outward sign, because anointing was also used to signal that one's legal and social status had been elevated outside of the tabernacle as well as inside of it. The men may have even anointed each other.

The act of anointing a person to accept the role of the priesthood did not guarantee they would become a prophet. Only God could anoint them with the Spirit of a true prophet. However, we do find one example when Elijah anointed Elisha to succeed himself as a prophet (1 Kings 19:16). Anointing with oil was still only a portrait of what the Spirit of God desired to perform in the lives of the priests, prophets, kings, and even the persistent faithful. Not every king or priest who was anointed lived in the fullness of the Spirit and did what was right before the Lord.

So what other criteria is there for being a prophet? To answer that question, we need to keep searching the Bible.

Moses had a sister, Miriam, and a brother, Aaron, who were also described as prophets. One day Miriam and Aaron spoke against Moses because he had taken a Cushite woman to be his wife. After their complaint, God spoke to Aaron and Miriam and explained that prophets are known by their dreams and visions, but Moses was more than this—he was so faithful he spoke to God face to face (Numbers 12:1-8). We can conclude from this illustration that dreams, visions, and even reciprocal communication (which we call "prayer") with God makes one a prophet. Afterword, God struck Miriam with leprosy and she became white and had to leave camp for seven days until God healed her. Zipporah, Moses' wife, was from the land of Cush or Ethiopia and could have been a black African woman (Numbers 12:10). That should give us all something to think about.

The original recipe for the holy anointing oil compound required liquid myrrh and olive oil as the base ingredients in this compound (Exodus 30:23-25). Frankincense and myrrh are both oleo gum resins which have an alcohol-soluble resin and water-soluble gum that can be extracted by grinding. The other ingredients used in this oil were most likely powdered cinnamon bark, powdered cassia leaves, and dried, powdered calamus root. All of these would have been combined in olive oil and macerated or heated until the plant compounds were dissolved and their properties were released into the oil. Then they could have been strained through a finely woven linen to filter out the plant pulp, left to sit, and had the top part of the oil poured off to purify it.

There are no written specifics, so we can only speculate how the anointing oil was made by the priests, which is described as *"the work of a perfumer"* (Exodus 30:25 [ESV]; 1 Chronicles 9:29).

King Solomon referred to myrrh and frankincense as *"powders of the merchants"* (Song of Solomon 3:6). It is logical that dried, ground plant powders would have also been preferred, because it was the best form in which to transport plant materials that traveled from such a great distance. The priests were in charge of making sure the oil and the incense did not become unclean or contaminated in any way, all according to the Hebraic law. Their merchants would have also understood Israel's demand for "clean" plant and animal products.

Details about the utility vessels used by the priests for their daily work are found in the Biblical books of Leviticus, Numbers, and a variety of other places. However, there is never mention of a "holy still or distillery" which would have been required for the priests to make essential oils through the process of steam distillation. It is probably not reasonable to think that this whole compound was made from essential oils. At the same time the translation of "*liquid myrrh*" (Exodus 30:23) might still be considered to be an EO by some because the earliest people known to have been distilling herbs and flowers to make perfumes during this time were on the island of Cyprus in the city of Pyrgos, dating back 4000 years.[8] This makes perfumery one of the oldest recorded occupations.

Consecrating the temple would have involved careful cleaning and polishing of each altar, vessel, plate and utensil by hand. Some of these vessels described would have been used for preparing the holy anointing oil itself. In the courtyard outside of the tabernacle, the priests also anointed the Basin and the Altar of Burnt Offering. These two altars also had utility vessels like pans for baking the unleavened wafer bread, pitchers for pouring, bowls for collecting blood, and tongs needed for the meat dissections and moving charcoal. All of these would have also been anointed.

During the consecration of the priests, first they consecrated the tabernacle and then the fragrant anointing oil was poured on the subjects' head and allowed to drip down onto their body which was clothed with the sacred linen garment (Exodus 29:7; Leviticus 8). A common vessel for pouring oil from was a horn, and later we read a that "flask" of oil was used. With the priests' consecration, as with the temple's consecration, blood and oil were used to represent the forgiveness of the priest's sin and for the mitigation of his guilt. Along with sprinkling the sacrificial blood, the anointing priest would also take the blood

---

[8] Belgiorno, M.R., *The Perfume of Cyprus, Third Revised Edition*, 2017. https://www.academia.edu/34788906/the_perfume_of_cyprus_revised_edition (Accessed 1-07-2020).

and use his thumb and finger to wipe it on the subjects' ear lobe, thumb, and big toe for a sin offering.

Why was the blood placed on these three specific parts of the body? Possibly because they represent the need to hear and know the law; the need to make contact with the Son of Man who came to live within their grasp (thumb); and the need to be anointed by the Spirit with *"beautiful feet"* for advancement of the Word (Romans 10:15). Can you picture the priest with blood, dripping from these areas, standing there as a visual image so the priest's might understand the forgiveness of past, present and even their future sins?

Consecration of priests appeared to be a prophetic act, as a copy and a shadow for what was to come in the future of Israel. That future was Jesus! After His arrest, the Roman guards used a barbed whip to scourge Him. This spattered Jesus' blood and would have left Him stripped of his skin and pierced in many places.

So let's ask ourselves, "What did the tabernacle (where God dwells), the priest's sin, and the linen garment sprinkled with the sacrificial blood and the fragrant oil come to mean with God's depiction of the everlasting covenant with Israel? The disciples taught us that the blood of Christ was shed for all our sins, and the Spirit anoints us with the oil of joy in our salvation.

> *Indeed, under the law almost everything is purified with blood, and without the shedding of blood there is no forgiveness of sin* (Hebrews 9:21 ESV).

The place where God dwelt with the Israelites was fearfully and wonderfully designed so they could recognize God's One and only Son when He came to them. Today we see God's accomplishments within the function and treatment of the tabernacle as a forerunner of what God has already done for us, in Jesus.

For on this day shall atonement be made for you to cleanse you. You shall be clean before the Lord from all your sins (Leviticus 16:30 ESV).

Myrrh and the Altar of Burnt Offering

The word used in Hebrew for burnt offering "*olah*" means going up in smoke or ascending offering.[xxvii] The Altar of Burnt Offering was made of acacia wood and was covered with bronze. It sat outside in the temple courtyard. It was in effect a large grill and, like the Altar of Incense, it had four horns, (one on each corner).

Day by day, two-year-old lambs were sacrificed on this altar: one in the morning with oil, wine, and flour, and one in the evening. On the Sabbath day two more lambs were sacrificed, two in the morning and again in the evening (Numbers 28:9-10). The sacrifice for the Sabbath day may have been completed by a second priest who was not required to enter the tabernacle that morning. It is possible at twilight, two actions occurred almost simultaneously: one priest would be preparing to sacrifice the first and then the second lamb, while a second priest was washing his hands in the Basin in order to enter the Holy Room, where he would light the incense and snuff out the lamps.

Was it coincidental that Jesus was on trial and condemned two times for his crimes and that Pilot washed his hands of it?

Jesus' trial by the High Priest Caiaphas took place early in the morning at dawn, when the rooster crowed. Caiaphas charged Jesus with blasphemy, which was punishable by death according to the Hebraic law, but not Roman law. Because of that limitation, Jesus was led to Pilate at the Roman Governor's headquarters in the sixth hour or 6 O'clock (John 19:14). Pilate questioned Jesus about His claims that He was the King of the Jews. Why? Because claiming to be a king under Roman law was punishable by death, and Caesar was the only recognized king. Pilate could not see that Jesus was a threat, so he publicly (and literally) washed his hands of the whole thing. Strangely, though, then he allowed Jesus to be prosecuted, making this the second time that Jesus - our Sacrificial Lamb - was tried and condemned (Matthew 27:24; John 18-19:14).

The prophet Isaiah himself may have already been anointed as priest when he acknowledged that God had anointed him. How did Isaiah describe his anointing? With the Spirit of joy, when he proclaimed the good news to the poor and released those who were brokenhearted, all with a wonderful thing called the "oil of gladness" (Isaiah 61:1-3 paraphrased).

Isaiah also realized his own sin and inadequacies. He had a vision of the Lord and wrote, *"Woe is me!" I cried. For I am a man of unclean lips"* (Isaiah 6:5 ESV). As Isaiah confessed his sin, and the sins of the people an angel of the Lord flew to him holding tongs and a live glowing coal taken from the altar. With it, the angel touched his mouth and claimed, *"See, this has touched your lips; and your guilt is taken away and your sin atoned for"* (Isaiah 6:7 ESV). This live coal would have come from the Altar of Burnt Offering where the Levite priests cooked the meat with the fat as a fragrant offering, and then they ate the meat as the portion of their inheritance.

The covenant law required them to save the blood and fat for God. The blood was used for ceremonial cleansing for the forgiveness of sin, while the fat was burned on the altar as a pleasing aroma. This was to be as an everlasting ordinance (Leviticus 3:17).

Although the task of cleaning and anointing all of the articles must have become repetitive and even boring, they were not optional. Animal sacrifice would have created the greatest amount of unpleasant work. Cleaning this altar would have taken a great deal of physical labor and time. The brass grill would have been cleaned with some kind of cleansing powder (Job 9:30 NIV) and then rubbed with the holy oil, which was fragrant and sanitizing.

The priests would have naturally enjoyed some of the tasks more than others. It appears these tasks were chosen by lot, like drawing straws to determine what daily work they would perform (Luke 1:9). That may have help to eliminate any complaints about doing any of the required work for that day.

God told Isaiah that Israel needed to stop bringing Him meaningless offerings. They were meaningless because their hands were full of blood, when they denied justice and ignored the fatherless and the widows (Isaiah 1:13-15). God also gave them some very good news, when He inspired King David to write:

> *Though your sins are like scarlet, they shall be as white as snow* (Isaiah 1:18 ESV).

The Romans and myrrh at the cross

Jesus had many close friends, but He also experienced what it was like to have enemies and knew that some people in the fringes of the crowd, who had proclaimed Him as the Prince of Peace, and had laid palm branches in His path only a few days earlier, might be persuaded to turn on Him and demand His crucifixion.

Jesus also knew He would rise from the dead and be restored to life everlasting. So over the past three years of Jesus' teaching of the disciples, He had tried to prepare them for the day He would be crucified. Just a few hours before His arrest, He had eaten the Passover meal in the upper room and explained to the disciples one last time that He must suffer and die in Jerusalem.

When the disciples were on the Mount of Olives before Jesus' arrest by the chief priest and the Roman guards, Jesus prayed. He asked His heavenly Father, *"that if it were possible, the hour might pass from him"* (Mark 14:35 ESV). While Jesus waited, He knew full well the excruciating pain He would endure. The prophet Isaiah described a suffering servant who was *"disfigured beyond recognition"* (Isaiah 52:14 NIV). The images we have all seen of Jesus on the cross do not even come close to the horror of His actual appearance.

During His crucifixion, Jesus suffered like any other man would have under these conditions. He would have experienced horrific physical pain; a deep emotional depression; the trauma of rejection; the humiliation of being falsely accused, hated, and misunderstood; and to add injury to injury, even abandonment by His own disciples. We may have all experienced these reactions at one time or another, but usually not to the point of our total desolation and death.

Wine mixed with myrrh was offered up to Jesus on the cross (Mark 15:23). From this passage in Mark, we know that myrrh was infused in wine or vinegar for medicinal purposes and was somehow supplied to the Romans for this purpose. This was most likely a common medication also used by others in their region as well.

Slow infusion (or maceration) of fresh herbs or powdered resin occurs when they are added to a liquid like wine-vinegar or oil and allowed to sit for up to six weeks. To speed up this process, the mixture can be cooked on low heat for four to six hours, and then strained. Then this liquid can either be reinfused to make it stronger, or simply used like it is.

Jesus suffered for about six hours on the cross (Mark 15). According to Mark's testimony, darkness covered the land, an appropriate response from creation when its creator was being murdered. Jesus chose to ware our shame and nakedness, even though He was without sin, and guilt or any wrongdoing.

> *So shall he sprinkle many nations. Kings shall shut their mouths because of him* (Isaiah 52:15 ESV).

As Jesus hung on the cross, some people in the crowd shouted that if He was the Messiah, He should have the power to come down and save Himself, especially after all of the miracles they had seen Him perform on the behalf of others (Mark 15:30). They did not understand Jesus had the power to do what they demanded, but that He would instead remain willing and faithful to fulfill the purpose for His life, to suffer in place of you and me.

Near the end, a Roman guard offered Jesus a drink of wine infused with myrrh. Although this would have been a nontoxic medicine in those days, it would not have been very effective at easing or preventing the suffering and agony of a gruesome crucifixion. But it was the only thing they had to offer Him. However, Jesus deliberately refused to drink this bitter and largely ineffective drink. He chose to suffer completely, with nothing to mitigate His pain, and then He cried out:

> *And now, Father, glorify me in your presence with the glory that I had with you before the world existed* (John 17:5 ESV).

When I inhale the sharp, balsamic, medicinal fragrance of myrrh, I remember my own personal need to be maintained as a vessel that can be used by God. Someday I will be made pure and radiant for the kingdom of God; but until then, day by day I require cleansing in the Word and the correcting serum of the Holy Spirit.

$$\approx A\Omega \approx$$

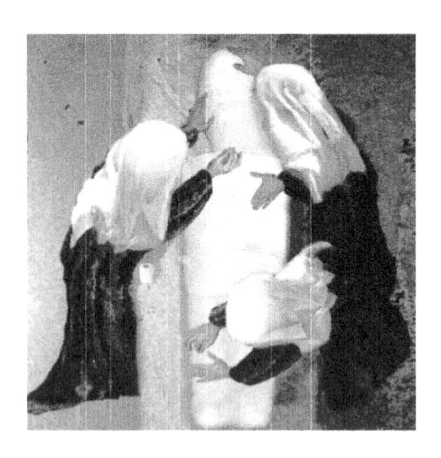

Chapter 6

Cinnamon, Cassia, and Calamus in the Holy Anointing Oil

Make a fragrant offering of cinnamon

Use cinnamon bark whole, or as an EO diluted at 1% in a carrier oil. Do not use *Cinnamonmum cassia* and *Acorus calamus*. Burn a cinnamon candle. Cinnamon is not recommended in a diffuser. Instead consider baked goods, cinnamon gum or candy sweetened with stevia or Xylitol. These are sweeteners from leaves or trees.

Plant name for cinnamon: *Cinnamomum zeylanicum* Family: Lauraceae. From India, Sri Lanka, and SE Asia and is now grown in Zanzibar and Indonesia as well. Note: Cinnamon has been in demand since the Egyptians and perhaps earlier. Ceylon or Sri Lanka were growing cinnamon when they were occupied by the Portuguese in 1536, the Dutch in 1656 and the English East India Company in 1796.[xxviii] Cinnamon became tremendously valuable, and was a large part of the "spice trade" that dominated that part of the world for centuries.

Oil extraction/characteristics: The bark, leaves, and roots are all used to make EO's. The bark is steam distilled by cohobation, a process of repeated distillation.[xxix] The leaves and roots are all extracted separately and used for different reasons. The oil is a yellow to brownish-yellow liquid. Cinnamon sticks are the bark of the tree that have been rolled up and dried. It does not kill the tree to remove the bark, and it is able to grow back. Cinnamon bark powders were most likely used for making the anointing oil.

Aroma: Not everyone has the same olfactory receptors for detecting fragrances. For some, cinnamon smells sweet, warm, spicy, woody, and very aromatic; others might describe the same batch of cinnamon as musty, sweet, and sharp.[xxx]

Emotional benefits: Cinnamon can be used for depressed people who are trapped in melancholia. Cinnamon has been reported to revitalize those suffering from nervous depression[xxxi] One might consider adding powdered cinnamon into coffee or tea before brewing or baking with it. It can also be added to shakes. Even burning it in a healthy candle is a good way to reap its fragrance.

Safety: Diffusing EO is not recommended. The use of cinnamon EO is not recommended for amateurs, because it should be pretested and the client interviewed to determine its safety. Cinnamon, calamus, and cassia are toxic when concentrated in the form of essential oils and can cause allergic reactions. Cinnamon is a skin irritant and the essential oil should not be used on the skin without diluting it to 1%, with a carrier oil like coconut or sunflower oil.

Cinnamon is not typically put into cosmetics or used on the skin because it is sensitizing and drying. If used over time it could cause the appearance of aging. However cinnamon is beneficial for gums and is frequently added to toothpaste. If you have even one allergy, you are at risk for developing other allergies, so be careful. Always use EO in bottles with an "orifice reducer" which is a plastic cap that provides one metered drop of oil at a time.

Cassia and *calamus* also part of the Anointing Oil, are actually hazardous essential oils.[xxxii] *Calamus* essential oil has cancer-causing agents. *Cassia* or Chinese cinnamon essential oil is sensitizing, meaning it can also cause allergies.

The European Union regulates how aromatherapists use essential oils. Why? Because they are up to 100 times stronger than the plants. Countries that regulate professional aromatherapists do not license them to dispense EO for internal use. In European countries, some physicians prescribe the use of essential oils. Medical doctors are able to determine their effectiveness, to recommend dosage, and to screen for toxicity. The FDA in the US does not regulate EO's or recognize them as a valid prescription for medical usage. In the US there is no other regulating body on the federal or state level. Although some are working toward getting this put into place.

The National Association for Holistic Aromatherapy (NAHA) and the International Federation of Professional Aromatherapists (IFPA) are independent organizations that advocate for training, education, and provide a certification, that is not recognized by most states.

Another way anyone can benefit from the oils plants make is to simply use more fresh herbs in your diets. Almost everyone can plant, grow, and learn to cook with aromatic herbs. This does not require a certification and although there is still some risk of an allergic reaction it is very low.

Biblical references for cinnamon, calamus and cassia

- Cinnamon along with myrrh in the holy anointing oil for sanctification and dedication of the altars and their vessels for worship.
- Cinnamon, cassia and calamus were required as a gift or a tithe for the tabernacle and later the temples.

- King David wrote a psalm about a righteous God who anoints with the oil of joy and whose garments smell of myrrh, aloes, and cassia (Psalms 45:7-8).
- King Solomon described cassia and cinnamon as attributes of his bride (Song of Solomon 4:13).
- Ezekiel wrote that cassia and calamus were used to barter for other goods (Ezekiel 27:19).
- Cinnamon has been found in Egyptian mummies, and could have been used for embalming Jacob and Joseph after they died in Egypt.

Historical application of cinnamon

Diodorus Sisculus, a Greek historian who died in c. 30 BC, described the use of myrrh, cedarwood oil, and cinnamon to prepare the body for burial. The leaf and the bark of the cinnamon tree were historically used for different medicinal benefits. Scripture does not distinguish which part of the plant was tithed for the tabernacle, but we assume it was the bark, as it is more aromatic.

Cinnamon is a strong antimicrobial, antifungal, and vermifuge, meaning it destroys parasites. It is also anesthetic, antiseptic, antibacterial and antispasmodic. It can also be used as a stimulant and insecticide.[xxxiii]

As with all plant life, the aroma and effectiveness of the plants vary from year to year and batch to batch, all depending on the condition of the soil and the amount of rainfall during that harvest year. Moses instructed the Israelites to bring the finest and best grade they could find for their tithe or gifts to the tabernacle. The lesson for us? There will always be something that competes for first place in our lives. Anything that distracts us from bringing God our best affects the quality of our relationship with Him, and may potentially become an idol and replace Him altogether.

Cinnamon and the bronze basin

Calamus, cassia and cinnamon would have all come into the Bible lands along the Grain Road, which was later called the "Silk Road."

These three plants would have been the most expensive components in the oil, worth significantly more than olive oil and myrrh. God instructed Moses in the use of these same plants for use in making the holy anointing oil for the consecration of the temple articles. It took Moses and Aaron seven days to complete the consecration of the tabernacle after its construction (Leviticus 8:35). This means that they would have observed a Day of Rest before this task was completed. This act of anointing and consecrating not only designated the temple items as holy and set aside specifically for worship, but also helped to purify them from bacteria and parasites.

Each utensil, dish, pot, vessel, fire pan, shovel, snuffer, and others would have been routinely cleaned along with the altars (2 Kings 25:14). In the courtyard was the bronze basin which sat on a brass stand and was used by the priest for washing his hands and feet before the he could enter the tabernacle. The priest understood from the covenant that law if he entered the tabernacle without washing, he would die (Exodus 30:21; 1 Kings 7:23-26). The basin held fresh, clean water, which would have been replaced daily. Polishing the basin with anointing oil would have helped to keep the basin and the water from growing bacteria, fungi and parasites as it sat open to the elements and the sunlight in the courtyard.

In King Solomon's temple there was a massive bronze washing basin called the Sea. It sat on top of 12 bronze sculptures of oxen, placed in groups of four facing north, south, east, and west. There were also ten smaller bronze basins and 100 other basins used in the courtyard (1 Kings 7; 2 Chronicles 4:8). The Sea was destroyed and the pieces taken to Babylon after the siege of Jerusalem (2 Kings 25:13). Cleansing the Altar of Burnt Offering and all of these basins with an anti-parasitic and antimicrobials found in the anointing oil may have also been crucial, because the priests were required to handle the blood. The act of anointing could have provided some protection for the priests' hands from bloodborne pathogens that are often found in animal blood.

Jacob and Joseph lived—and died—in Egypt

Ancient Egyptians also used cinnamon, myrrh, and many other types of fragrant plant materials during this same time to embalm and "mummify" their dead. The Israelite and Egyptian cultures became entwined because of their close proximity and approximately 400 years of being subjected as slaves there.

Abraham, Isaac, and Jacob were the founding fathers of the Israelite tribes. Jacob had twelve sons. His son Joseph was the oldest of two sons born to Rebekah, the wife whom Jacob loved most. After Jacob had lived in Egypt for 17 years he died, and Joseph had him embalmed. We presume this was an Egyptian embalming with spice and linen wrappings; however, this would not have included the mutilation of the corpse for which the ancient Egyptians were known.

Before Jacob died, he blessed his twelve sons, and those specific blessings were recorded. To his fourth son Judah, he spoke a prophecy about One who would come out of his tribe. This would be a remarkable person who would gather the people, and whose garments would be washed in the blood of grapes (Genesis 49:10-11). After Jacob had been embalmed, Joseph took his father's bones home to Canaan and buried him in the land where Joseph's great-grandfather Abraham and Grandfather Isaac were also buried.

Before Joseph's death, he had the Israelites take an oath and promise to take his bones back to Canaan when they left Egypt. Why? Because he had faith that God would return the Israelites to his family's land. After Joseph died, like his father Jacob he was also embalmed and eventually returned to Canaan.

After Jacob's and Joseph's burial in Egypt, the use of spice and linen wrappings may have become acceptable for the Israelites to use. Research of Egyptian mummies have revealed that they used a lot of different plant preparations to mummify their dead. It seems like they used what they had available, or perhaps more likely what people could afford to pay. Cinnamon would have been costly, but pine resin and cedarwood would have been more affordable.

We cannot be sure what went into the embalming of Jacob and then Joseph, but it is possible cinnamon was used. Burials with linen and spices would have been possible only for those who could afford it, therefore, it was reserved for kings or for the wealthy, which would have included Joseph and his family (Isaiah 53:9; Matthew 27:57-60).

Sometime after this, the Israelites became enslaved by another Pharaoh, who would not let them return to their homeland, but God had a plan to break their chains in Egypt.

After God freed the Israelite slaves, they wandered in the desert for 40 years unable to live by faith and with a lot of grumbling. Living in the desert they would have become familiar with the caravan routes which were coming and going north to Babylon and Assyria, and south to Egypt. These routes would have also provided them with a way to sell or trade goods like spices, sheep, goats, handmade items, and (sadly) even servants like Joseph.

King Solomon wrote about an adulterous woman who perfumed her bed with myrrh, aloes, and cinnamon. Since we know these fragrances were also used for anointing a corpse, one has to wonder if Solomon was illustrating how her actions would lead to the death and burial of those who came under her power. When sin is left to reign, it will eventually result in one's spiritual or physical death (Proverbs 7:17-27).

Myrrh, aloes, and spice

There is nothing in the Bible about the process for making the anointing compound for the dead. So it is also plausible that many other spices not specifically recorded in the Bible could have been used. Many households would have used local herbs for their own medical purposes. Cinnamon and cassia from China and calamus from India would have been less common and more expensive, but many other herbs were local.

There are two different types of aloes mentioned in the Bible. The first of these plants is thought to have been the *Aloe vera,* plant which is a succulent from the *Liliaceae* family. This plant has a long history of being farmed and used for pharmaceuticals. It has a thick gel-like pulp inside its heavy, fleshy leaves that is thought to have healing benefits for skin.

There were also *lign aloes* or aloe-woods that were valued during this time as well (Numbers 24:6). The Egyptians would have also used this wood for embalming their Pharaohs and they would have had many ways to mix them. They also embalmed cats, birds, alligators and other creatures they worshiped as gods.[xxxiv]

King Solomon also wrote about frankincense, myrrh, and aloe trees (Song of Songs 4:14). There are several aromatic woods that may have been aloes. For instance, *Santalum album*, called "sandalwood," and *Aquilaria malaccenis,* called "agarwood," which is an aromatic evergreen tree.[xxxv] Both of these trees are on the *Red List* as vulnerable and critically endangered species. Agarwood grows sparsely in Asia and Malaysia and has a woody, fruity, vanilla, musk-like fragrance. Sandalwood is primarily from India and South East Asia and has a musty, woody, base note that lingers. Today there are also new sandalwood farms in Australia which were started to supply woods for essential oils. Both of these trees are on the *Red List* as vulnerable and critically endangered species. Agarwood grows sparsely in Asia and Malaysia and has a woody, fruity, vanilla, musk-like fragrance. Sandalwood is primarily from India and South East Asia and has a musty, woody, lingering base note. There are also new sandalwood farms in Australia that were started specifically to supply woods for essential oils.

Perfumers may have blended the embalming spices in Israel, as there is no evidence that the priests did this. Myrrh and cinnamon could have been ground down into a fine powder and added to acacia gum (which was as an adhesive). Fragrant sawdust from the aloe trees could have been macerated or heated with olive oil and possibly strained or used as a thick paste for topical application. This kind of substance would need to be stored in clay jars with a wide mouth so one could reach into the jar and retrieve the substance by hand. Then it could have been applied directly onto a corpse, as well as over the first layers of the linen closest to the body. Many of us in the west associate funerals with the scent of roses. The ancients would have had a different fragrant association for funerals with: sweet aloe woods, myrrh, and even cinnamon.

Jesus and His disciples ate their last meal at the end of the Passover week and Jesus was arrested very early in the morning and crucified. He died a few hours before the special Passover Sabbath began, and Joseph of Arimathea and Nicodemus were granted permission by the Roman officials to take His body down for burial. Jesus was in the tomb (as he had predicted) for three days and three nights.

In the Gospel of John, we read that strips of linen were used according to the Jewish burial traditions, but very little can be found in Scripture about this particular tradition. Nothing in the laws of Moses defines burial requirements or traditions, possibly because God thought it was more important how the Israelites were to live their lives rather than how they were to be buried. Caves were purchased or used for burials, and on occasion we read that people were buried in the land of their inheritance (Joshua 24:30). We also know from Scripture that it was considered a curse to be left on the ground with no burial (Deuteronomy 28:26).

So after Jesus' body was removed from the cross, Joseph of Arimathea and Nicodemus loosely wrapped Jesus with linen and laid Him in a new tomb with 75 pounds (33 kilos or one talent) of myrrh and aloes, which happened to be the same weight as the solid gold lampstand in the tabernacle (John 19:39). The weight of the lampstand also brings into mind a parable Jesus told to the multitudes: how the light from a city on a hill will not be hidden, but rather it is raised up on a stand so that everyone in the house may see (Matthew 5:14).

Jesus' crucifixion would have deeply affected those closest to Him, as there was no doubt they were overwhelmed with sadness and grief. The load of spice involved in his burial, with its heavy, wood, musk-like, vanilla, fruity fragrance would have lingered in the memories of everyone involved with this excruciating event.

While the Romans would have been busy sealing up the tomb and getting the guards in position to protect the area from tampering, the people would have returned to their homes. Once again, all labor ceased as the Israelite community began Havdalah, when they would remain quarantined in His rest. Jesus' body rested in a fragrant tomb at the end of the Passover-Week on the Sabbath Day, one of the most important holy days in Israel.

> *You have loved righteousness and hated wickedness. Therefore God, your God, has anointed you with the oil of gladness beyond your companions; your robes are all fragrant with myrrh and aloes and cassia* (Psalms 45:7-8 ESV).

Do you recall the variety of meanings for Shabbat or Sabbath rest?

- to ensoul
- a pleasing fragrance
- an appetite
- to yearn

- inner passion or joy
- inner being

Now we understand! From the beginning of creation our All-Knowing Father had this in His plan *as a copy and a shadow of heavenly things.* We are still surrounded, endowed, encased by a passionate loving Creator God who desires to make Himself known to us.

In three days and the resurrection

Early in the morning on the first day of the week (which was Sunday for Israel), the women closest to Jesus set out for the tomb where Jesus was laid. Their intention was to finish anointing His body with more spice (Mark 16:1-2). Depending on the way the word "spice" is used in the Hebrew language, it may also mean a blend of different spices. This means that we do not know how many different spices the women brought in addition to those which were already there.

When the women set out, it may have been about the same time the shopkeepers would have been setting up for the day. The marketplace in Jerusalem would have been packed with travelers, which would have made it an energized location for the events which had just taken place. Over baskets of zesty, fragrant and colorful spices commonly used as the local drug store as well as for cooking the local cuisine, men and women would have begun to exchange their accounts of what had happened to Jesus on the cross.

When the women arrived at the open tomb, it would have still been pungent with the aromatic spices. When they looked inside and discovered that Jesus' body was missing, one can imagine their amazement and their questions!

It was there that they encountered the angel of the Lord, who announced to them that Jesus had risen from the dead (Luke 24:4-6)! As the women began to understand what this meant, a great surge of relief and joy came over them as the Words

Jesus had spoken "anointed" their spirits with a whole new meaning. A thousand years before Jesus' death and resurrection King David wrote this Psalm:

> *Therefore my heart is glad and my tongue rejoices; my body also will rest secure, because you will not abandon me to the realm of the dead, nor will you let your faithful one see decay* (Psalm 16:10 NIV).

On the third day, that awesome Sunday, the news that Jesus' tomb was open and *empty* would have resonated through the marketplace. Some people even came to the markets with unfathomable reports that the tombs of dead saints were opened, and that those dead had risen and appeared to them! (Matthew 27:52).

The people would have been asking many questions: Would the Roman guards be executed for losing track of Jesus' body, or would the authorities pay them off to tell a lie? Could Jesus have been the Messiah, The Anointed One, Israel had been waiting for? Many people witnessed Jesus hanging on the cross, yet now there were reports that this dead man had been seen alive. Could Jesus be the *"King of the Jews"* like the Roman guards had facetiously written in Aramaic and nailed to a plaque on His cross?

Over the next forty days, Jesus appeared to the disciples and taught them about the Kingdom of God. He even ate with them (Luke 24:42-43). He also intentionally appeared to over 500 people at one time to be sure there was no doubt He had risen to life! (1 Corinthians 15:6)

Can you imagine the rumors in the marketplace? These would have passed from person to person and back again for forty days, as each person heard about what was taking place. After forty days had passed, Jesus ascended into the heavens, but with a promise that He would return when His heavenly Father decided the time was right (Luke 21:25-28).

The parallels are stunning. In three days, God spoke, and the earth brought forth its plants and herbs yielding their seeds and oils, and it was good. In three days, Jesus rose from the dead and this was even better news. Even creation itself appears to be a *copy and a shadow of heavenly things.*

When I take in the sweet, warm, spicy, woody fragrance of cinnamon, it reminds me to keep some things holy, special, or sacred in my life. The heat and spice from cinnamon helps me recall the work the priests did in the tabernacle to keep each vessel and the altars themselves purified and serviceable. When we are a clean (forgiven) vessel the Spirit may also anoint us with gifts of joy, visions, prophecy, guidance, discernment, teaching, miracles, giving, and healing for the common good of the church (Acts 2:17, 8:29; 1 Corinthians 12:1-11; Romans 15:13).

> *Now it is God who makes both us and you stand firm in Christ. He anointed us, set his seal of ownership on us, and put his Spirit in our hearts as a deposit, guaranteeing what is to come* (2 Corinthians 1:21 NIV).

≈ AΩ ≈

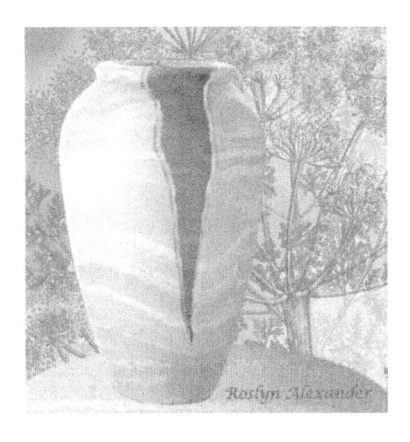

Chapter 7

Mary Anointed Jesus with Spikenard

The fragrant offering of nard

Spikenard or *Nardostachys jatamansi* with the common name "nard." Nard is on the Red List as critically endangered (CR).

Family: Valerianaceae.

Substitute: When one substitutes spikenard with vetiver it has almost the same aroma and benefits. You may also use fresh ginger root as a visual and fragrant aid. Nard is a flowering plant with pink blooms, like those found on the cover. Small pink carnations are a similar looking flower that you might even consider using as a display to tell the story of Mary. If you desire to make a perfume try blending vetiver along with, geranium rose, mandarin orange, and 1 drop of ylang ylang in a carrier oil at 3-5% for a fragrant offering or perfume oil.

Plant name: Chrysopogon zizanioides, or vetiver. Family: Poaceae or Gramineae from a family of bunchgrass, something like lemongrass. Vetiver is a tall perennial grass grown to prevent soil erosion. It is found in India, Sri Lanka, and Malaysia. Both vetiver and spikenard have an aromatic rhizome root like the ginger plant. Both of these plants are native to the Himalayan region of India.[xxxvi] Both of them may be dwindling, so keep checking the *Red List* for new developments.

Oil extraction/characteristics: Steam distilled from dried crushed root. This is a thick heavy oil that is slow to drop from the bottle's orifice reducer. It typically requires warming with the hand or in warm water.

Aroma: Vetiver has a sweet, well-rounded, spicy, woody, and slightly camphor-like aroma. Spikenard's aroma is heavy, sweet, woody, and herbaceous or musk-like. Vetiver, like spikenard is a base note. Many prefer the fragrance of vetiver over that of spikenard essential oil, because it is lighter but still very fragrant.

Emotional benefits: Some people use nard to find their inner balance, soothing, rejuvenating, and sedating. Its effects are similar to the root of the valerian plant.[xxxvii]

Biblical references for anointing and nard

- King Solomon wrote about spikenard ("nard") in his book (Song of Solomon 1:12; 4:13):
- Nard was used to anoint Jesus for His burial (Matthew 26:6-13; Mark 14:3-9; Luke 7:36-50; John 12:3).
- Spikenard was used to make expensive perfumes reserved for the wealthy who could afford to lavish it on those they loved (Mark 14:3-9).
- The anointing of the Holy Spirit and baptism in the New Testament are at times used simultaneously (Matthew 3:11; Mark 1:8; Luke 3:16; Acts 1:5; 11:16).

Historical application of nard

Spikenard was useful for treating leprosy, a skin condition in which a bacterium that covers whole parts of the body appears with scaley white raised patches.[xxxviii] Nard is warming, drying and healing to wounds or ulcers that seep. Dioscorides wrote that nard is also good for nausea, indigestion, menstrual problems, inflammations and conjunctivitis.[xxxix]

When substituting with vetiver, it can be used to encourage forgiveness, reduce fearfulness, and to instill calm and balance.[xl] How interesting that some think a fragrance can help us to forgive! It is sad to say that most of us could find a reason to wear vetiver every day, but it is not until we put into action what Jesus taught, and we willingly take up our own cross, and forgive like Christ forgives us, that we can truly wear the heavenly fragrance of forgiveness (Matthew 6:14).

In Bible times the plant alcohols from herbs and oils became valuable for cosmetics as well as for personal hygiene. Nard would have been far too expensive for most people in those days to use for a deodorant or a medicine. Even a hand-carved, alabaster stone container would have been expensive, since glass was not made by the Romans until around 1 AD.

Nard's plant compounds are bactericidal, deodorant, and fungicidal, because of this it can literally help control the bad odor caused by bacteria that grow on our bodies. Learning to detect these odors used to play a bigger role in medicine than it does today, which is to our loss. There is a whole science devoted to uncovering how fragrant plant volatiles interact with malodourous bacteria, fungi, and even insects that sometimes also emit odors of their own. There are also other studies that explore the bioelectricity of plants which behave like they have a memory that has been an essential design for their adaptation and survival as the first living single cell organisms on our planet.

Detecting good bacteria in food is useful for making wine, beer or cheese and is also an ancient skill. Plant compounds in our food from fermentation may also alter mood, behavior, or our health in ways we do not always comprehend. This is not mystical, but it is rather how God designed us to receive chemicals and information about our environment through built-in olfactory pathways. Of course, God may also work outside of our life's normal order when He performs miracles.

The role of women in Israel

Daily work defined in the Torah (the first five books of the Bible written by Moses) created a culture that would have permeated Israel. It would also have been farther reaching as demands for "clean goods" and trade went well beyond Israel's borders.

The Torah also helped to define the roles of men and women in Israel. Women would have been involved in preparing and gathering tithes and offerings. They would have also ground wheat for the temple along with their own family's needs. We know from Scripture that there were also female prophets in the Old Testament. Sarah, Abraham's wife, is considered by some to be a prophet, because when the Pharaoh took her (inappropriately) to be his wife, even though she was already married to Abraham, a plague came upon his people (Genesis 12:12-20).

How had this come about? Abraham had been afraid that the Pharaoh would kill him and take Sarah for himself, because she was so beautiful. So he told Pharaoh that Sarah was his sister, which led to the Pharaoh taking her to be his wife, but God intervened. He acted on Sarah's behalf, and when Pharaoh's household became ill, he sent her back to Abraham. After that, Pharaoh's household recovered.

We have already mentioned that Miriam, Moses' sister, was a prophet but there were many others:

- Deborah, who led Israel in battle (Judges 4-5);
- Hannah, who gave birth to Samuel after she vowed to give her first born son to the temple (1 Samuel 1-2);
- Abigail, who became a wife to King David after demonstrating acts of bravery (1 Samuel 31);

Roslyn Alexander

- Huldah, who was raised up during a time of revival in Israel (2 Kings 22:14-20);
- Esther, a Persian Jew, who is considered to be a prophet by the Jews because she prevented their destruction in Persia by an evil man named Haman (the book of Esther);
- Isaiah also wrote about a woman prophet, but gave her no name (Isaiah 8:3);
- Anna was a prophet who lived at the temple, and who spoke to Mary and Joseph about baby Jesus as the *"redemption of Israel"* shortly after their encounter with another prophet named Simeon (Luke 2:36-38).

A prophet never acts on his or her own behalf, but instead is anointed by the Holy Spirit to speak, act, or intercede between God and His people.

One of the greatest prophets is a woman whom we rarely think of in that way: Mary, the mother of Jesus, who saw into the future of her Son and His work. Her dear cousin Elizabeth, who gave birth to John the Baptist, also prophesized about Mary's very special baby.

Moses' law does not define what worship should or should not look like for women at the tabernacle. After the construction of Solomon's temple, we are told that women could not enter the main courtyard, but were only permitted to pray inside a forecourt near the northern gate. Women in the Hebraic culture were considered unclean during their monthly issue of blood. This would no doubt have kept them from some social events in Israel, but I am sure that they had their own special meeting places with each other. Scripture does not tell us where in Herod's temple Anna was when she encountered Mary and Joseph. However, Josephus, a Jewish historian, described Herod's temple forecourt as having its own set of gates which were used by the women. Perhaps Anna the prophet met Mary there? [xli]

Quite often God led the prophets to perform actions that would make a hard-to-ignore point:

- Jeremiah smashed clay jars (1Jeremiah 9:10-13);

- Ezekiel laid on the ground bound in ropes and shaved his head (Ezekiel 4:1-8);
- The prophet Amos preached about immoral and unethical behavior when he warned the Israelites that God would punish them when they sold their poor into slavery for the price of sandals and cheated them out of food by selling the chaff with the wheat.
- The prophet Micah preached against those who cheat others with faulty scales and deceitful weights (Amos 4:1; 8:6; Micha 6:11).
- John the Baptist demanded that people repent from their sins, and when they did, he immersed them in water.

These prophets demonstrated that our actions do speak louder than words, especially when the Spirit moves us to act.

Consider Tabatha ("Dorcas" in Greek), who is called a disciple. She had spent hours making garments to clothe the needy in her community. After Tabatha suddenly died, Peter brought her back to life through the power of God (Acts 9:36).

There would have been many other acts by women that were not recorded. For example, Jesus told the parable about a widow who gave her last coin as a tithe, but I am sure other women who followed Jesus also helped to feed and care for the poor in their communities, and they were never mentioned. Women like Tabatha were also disciples of Christ, although they were not specifically named as such in the Scriptures.

After Jesus' resurrection and ascension, we come across a man named Philip, who served as one of the first deacons in the early church. A deacon was a man or woman who were Godly, and who demonstrated self-control when tested. They assisted with the Lord's Supper, facilitated collecting the offerings and helped settle disputes or conflicts so the Word could continue to be preached. They were also called servants of the church (Timothy 3:8-12; Romans 16:1).

Paul wrote that Philip had virgin daughters who prophesied, yet it's too easy to focus on how Paul asked these virgins to cover their heads. Even men covered their heads during prayer, and at other times for worship in the temple. What is significant here is that women and men were worshiping together, as if the church had already made a huge paradigm shift because of the teachings of Christ (Acts 21:9).

At times Jesus' interactions with women were seen as radical, even outrageous:

- He was witnessed talking alone to an alien Samaritan woman at the ancient well of Jacob (John 4:1-42).
- Jesus saved the life of the woman caught in adultery, when He challenged her accusers to cast the first stone if they were without sin, which of course none of them were (John 8:7).
- Jesus encouraged Mary and Martha to sit and listen to His teaching in their home instead of the usual preparing food or doing housework. By doing this He was extending to them the same rights as men had to sit, listen, and learn during a time when women typically had no formal training outside the home (Luke 10:38-42).

After Jesus' death on the cross, Mary Magdalene, Mary the mother of James, and Salome brought spices so they could finish anointing Jesus' body (Mark 16:1). It was more usual for this work to be done by women, in part because of the laws that defined clean and unclean, but this also gave women the honor of being the first to witness that Jesus was alive. So the last were the first (Matthew 20:16). Joanna and Susanna, two of the women who had helped support Jesus' ministry, were also among some of the first to receive the news of Jesus' resurrection (Luke 5:27).

These and many other women became vital to the growth of the early church. Junia and her husband, Andronicus, ended up in jail with Paul (Romans 16:7). Phoebe was a deaconess in the church at Cenchreae (Romans 16:6). Priscilla and her husband, Aquila, were co-workers with Paul as they risked their lives in the work of the early church. Lydia, who sold purple cloth, hosted Paul in her home (Acts 16:14). We understand from Scripture that women also acted using gifts that they received from the anointing of the Spirit in the early days of the church.

Mary and the anointing of Jesus for His burial

Matthew, Mark, Luke, and John all wrote about Mary (not the mother of Jesus), who anointed Jesus (Matthew 16:21, 26:6-10; Mark 14:3; Luke 7:37-50; 8:1-3; John 12:1-3). There are variations in these accounts, but if you read each one, you will realize that there are two separate places where this happened—and possibly with two different Mary's!

Luke, a physician and evangelist, wrote about a woman who was a sinner and who had been healed from seven unclean spirits (Luke 8:2). We do not understand exactly what this affliction might have been or if this affliction is still experienced today, but whatever it was she would have been extremely grateful to Jesus for healing her and making her whole again. Luke also wrote that she and some of the other women who had been healed were supporting Jesus and the disciples with their own money. This unnamed woman, who we will call "Mary," followed Jesus and the disciples. She would have witnessed Jesus teaching the disciples to pray and anoint the sick with oil, possibly in the very same way in which she had been healed (James 5:14; Luke 9:2; John 6:2; Acts 10:38).

As His destined time to die approached, Jesus prepared to return to Jerusalem for His last Passover. Mary, who had been healed, would have heard Jesus remind His disciples that He must suffer many things from the chief priests and elders, and that He would die, and on the third day would be raised to life. Mary would have begun to grieve because she knew she could trust Jesus at His word.

In her sorrow and out of her gratitude for what Jesus had done for her, Mary brought an exotic perfume, worth a year's wages, to anoint Jesus. She must have understood the earthly value of the perfume, and how it had come from the far east with merchants who had traveled into Jerusalem along the Grain Roads. This perfume may have been one of the most valuable items she owned. It could have even been part of her own dowry if she was married, but we know very little about her.

What we do understand is that, within her spirit, she became determined to anoint Jesus with her aromatic perfume. When Mary arrived at Simon's house Jesus was reclined at the table eating. This would have been on a Roman-style couch where Jesus would have laid on His left side and reached out with His right hand (the "clean" hand) for food that would have been presented on a table at the same height as the couch. This position allowed Jesus to stretch out with His feet at the end of the couch, at about knee-height to Mary. Mary would have stood leaning over Jesus' feet at the end of the couch with her long, dark hair falling down. She broke the waxy seal of the alabaster perfume bottle and poured it out as she anointed Jesus' feet.

Breaking the waxy, or resin seal may have had a deeper, cultural meaning that has been lost through time. Once the seal was broken, oxygen would enter the bottle and the plants' volatiles would be released from their entombment so the remaining perfume would break down more rapidly. All perfumes are dated even today but would have been even more so in Bible times. Why? The shelf life of a perfume would have been much shorter without modern containers, refrigeration, or additives (which are usually "impurities"). The woman wept at the thought of harm coming to Jesus, and as her tears fell on Jesus' feet, she used her hair to wipe her tears away. What a dramatic, emotional moment this must have been for everyone who was there!

Luke wrote that a Pharisee watching Mary thought to himself that if Jesus was a prophet, why would He let this woman, who is a "sinner", touch Him? Jesus turned to the Pharisee and could see his contempt for her. He told him a story about a moneylender who forgave a man with an enormous debt as well as a man with a lesser debt. What was His point? Jesus wanted to illustrate that her gratitude and gift had been in proportion to what she had been forgiven. He turned to Mary and explained to them,

Essence of Day

> *Therefore, I tell you, her many sins have been forgiven—as her great love has shown. But whoever has been forgiven little loves little* (Luke 7:36-50 NIV).

As Mary anointed Jesus' feet with the fragrant perfume, the plant volatiles that filled the room would have been sedating and calming for Jesus, Mary herself, and even the others in the room would have been sedated by as the heavy, sweet, woody, spice like aroma. The volatiles from spikenard in the air would have entered their lungs where these plant chemicals would have made their way into their bloodstream. Plant compounds like α-patchoulene and β-gurjunene are fat soluble and would have also passed through the epidermis and dermis layers of skin on Jesus' feet and into the palms of Mary's hands and into their bloodstreams as she applied the oil.

Mary anointed Jesus and her tears flowed because of her great love and gratitude for what He had done for her and for so many others. After which Jesus replied to Mary's critics with the shocking news that she had *"anointed Him for His burial"* (Mark 14:8 KJV). Many hours later, the fragrance in Mary's hair may have even lingered as she watched Jesus suffer and die.

For thousands of years the Israelite's worshiped with fragrant sacrificial offerings and fragrant anointing as part of their everlasting covenant to consecrate the temple for worship. Israel's prophets had written many times about the coming of the *Messiah,* which came from a root word *mashiach,* which interestingly means to massage with oil. The perfume oil Mary applied to Jesus would have been like the oil of sadness or mourning, but soon her mourning would be dissipated as she became anointed by the Spirit with joy (Isaiah 61:3).

Jesus, the Anointed One, who was conceived in the Spirit and born of flesh, did not require anointing like the temple priests, as He had already been consecrated from the moment of His conception to accomplish the will of His heavenly Father.

We do not know what happened to Mary after the ascension of Jesus, but we assume she would have continued to use her essential spiritual gifts of service and sacrificial giving during the formation of the early church (Acts 2:45). Men and women today still receive anointing of spiritual gifts, for the good of the church (1 Corinthians 12:9). Only with this anointing and transformation of the Holy Spirit are we able to break free from our own sin and death (Romans 12:2).

Pentecost and the anointing of the disciples

After Jesus rose from the dead, He met with the disciples at various times over the next 40 days, and taught them about the kingdom of God. Before Jesus ascended into the heavens, He instructed the disciples to fast, pray, and wait for the help from His Father (Acts 1:4). The disciples were obedient as they waited in the upper room doing all Jesus had instructed them to do.

The noises from the street below their room would have steadily increased until the arrival of the third most important annual holy day pilgrimage into Jerusalem. While the disciples were in the upper room, they would also have been counting down the last ten days of the seven weeks or 50 days from Passover when the holy day of Shavuot (Pentecost) would arrive.

The main reason for Pentecost was to commemorate the day on which Moses had presented the Torah to the Israelites. The counting between these two holy days was important because the Passover marked the time God gave them freedom from their bondage to slavery. At the same time, the covenant law offered them freedom from the bondage of sin by making them aware of their inward and outward sins against each other and their heavenly Father.

In order for them to fully receive the gift of the Torah, they would first need to know it, believe it was beneficial for their life and then remember to act on it. This holy day was combined with the grain harvest or the *Feast of Weeks*, because the word of God is also considered to be a first fruit from the Spirit. Followers of the faith from all over the area would gather their grains right from the threshing floor and take them directly to the temple.

When the day of Shavuot or Pentecost arrived it had been 50 days since Passover and ten days since the ascension of Christ. The disciples were fasting and praying in the upper room, when tongues of fire entered the room and settled on every one of them (Acts 2:1-4). Each disciple began to speak in foreign languages, as they moved out of the house and into the street to publicly proclaim all the magnificent acts that God had accomplished through His son Jesus. Many God-fearing Israelites were amazed to hear the Word of God in their own tongues, and this led to many of them to believe in this good news.

The church grew to three thousand on that single day in Jerusalem (Acts 2:41). Even a large number of the temple priests believed (Acts 6:7). The Holy Spirit baptized the disciples (or "immersed" them) so that they overflowed with the Spirit. With this powerful anointing, they joyfully proclaimed God's righteousness for the rest of their days.

The collective church today is still a product of this anointing from the Spirit, as it has inherited that which was provided at Pentecost. The prophet Isaiah wrote about the future glory of Israel when they would receive

> *the oil of gladness instead of mourning, the garment of praise instead of a faint spirit; that they may be called oaks of righteousness, the planting of the Lord, that he may be glorified* (Isaiah 61:3 ESV).

The apostles and disciples of Jesus were certainly trees of righteousness that God had intentionally planted, along with so many others throughout the history of Israel. Over thousands of years the Israelite priests, prophets, scribes and the patient faithful were inspired by the Holy Spirit to record 39 books of what we now call the "Old Testament" (but which does not mean that it isn't still important and applicable). After Jesus' ascension, the Holy Spirit also inspired the apostles and other followers to write 27 more letters and books of what we call the "New Testament." This gives us a Bible of 66 Books.

> *These are my words that I spoke to you while I was still with you, that everything written about me in the Law of Moses and the Prophets and the Psalms must be fulfilled."* (Luke 24:44 ESV).

Mary and the other women who sat under the teaching of Jesus also received gifts of the Spirit. Luke quoted Jesus when he wrote, *"In the same way those of you who do not give up everything they have cannot be my disciples"* (Luke 14:33 NIV). Certainly, Mary gave all she had. This raises an extremely important question. Are we holding back? Does the church today suffer in its actions and its use of spiritual gifts because we fail to give all we have?

Mary's case is sensational. Jesus made no mention of gender when He described the qualifications for being a disciple, so this amazingly included Mary. While materialism can still be an idol that quenches the Spirit, Mary quite possibly gave up the most valuable possession she owned when she poured it out on Jesus. What would we do if we were standing there by Jesus, holding a year's worth of wages in our hands?

The next time I am tempted to covet the exotic, heavy, sweet, woody, herbaceous, musk-like fragrance of spikenard, which is now endangered because of mankind's neglect, greed, and materialism, I will remember how Jesus honored and transformed Mary's life in the Spirit.

In pouring this ointment on my body, she has done it to prepare me for my burial. Truly, I say to you, wherever the gospel is proclaimed in the whole world, what she has done will also be told in memory of her (Matthew 26:12-13 ESV).

$$\approx A\Omega \approx$$

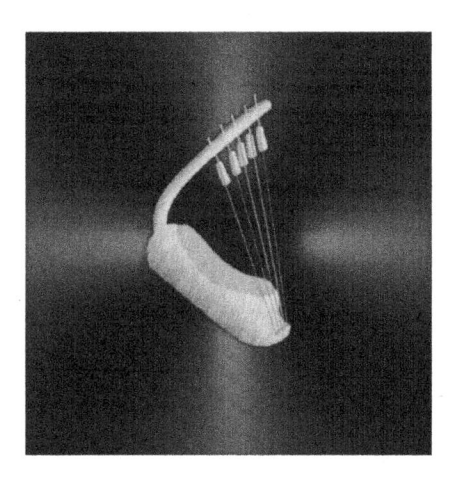

Chapter 8

Myrtle, Palms, Willows and Olive for the Festival of Booths

Make a fragrant offering of myrtle

Myrtle, palms, willows. You also might find value in presenting any of these as potted plants. Olive wood utensils or cups, baskets made from willow branches can also be used to illustrate this chapter. All of these plants are associated with peace in the Holy Lands along with the olive tree.

Plant name: Myrtus communis.

Family: Myrtaceae. Myrtle is a small evergreen tree or shrub with fragrant white-to-pink flowers, long, and sharp-pointed leaves, and red-brown bark. Myrtle is native to the Mediterranean and western Asia. The essential oil is currently produced in Tunisia, France, Corsica, Spain, Morocco and Italy.[xlii]

Oil extraction/characteristics: Steam distillation of leaves, stems, and sometimes the flowers. A mobile oil, yellow-to-orange, and sometimes green in color. The Greek Physician

Dioscorides (who died c. 90 AD) wrote that myrtle was good for lung and bladder infections.[xliii] It improves the immune system, as well as being an antiseptic, astringent and expectorant. It helps to decrease the production of mucus because of its anti-catarrhal properties.[xliv] Even head lice can be treated with myrtle.[xlv]

Emotional benefits: Myrtle is lightly sedative.[xlvi] The berries of the bush have been used to flavor food and drink, and have at times even been used to replace pepper. It was popular in Roman gardens as a hedge or decorative bush. Willow bark was used for medicinal purposes and contains acetylsalicylic acid used to make salicylic acid for pain relief but is not used for its fragrance.

Aroma: I have two bottles of myrtle. One is from Tunisia which smells fresh, herbaceous, sweet camphor-like, and a bit floral. The second bottle is from Morocco and is more herbaceous and camphor-like, with less floral. The aroma from myrtle changes somewhat depending on where it is grown. This is actually true with all plants and their oils to some degree, but seems to be exaggerated with myrtle, perhaps because it also grows in a wider variety of locations. Myrtle is a middle note. Some oils are also adulterated with other fragrant oils that are less expensive to boost or enhance sales.

Biblical references for myrtle and leafy woods

- Leafy woods like myrtle, willows, olive and palms are used for the celebration of Sukkot, or the Festival of the Booths (Leviticus 23).
- The Fest of Weeks begins in late May on our calendar and the Festival of the First Fruits ends the harvest season celebration along with Sukkot.
- A portion of the crops grown were again offered to the temple priests in baskets sometimes made from willow branches (Deuteronomy 26).
- Palm trees were carved into the walls of the Holy Room and the Most Holy Room of Solomon's temple (1 Kings 6:29).

Roslyn Alexander

- An unknown author of a Psalm wrote about Israel's capture by Babylon when they wept but were still required to sing and play their harps. They hung their harps in the willows and remembered Zion (Psalms 137:1-3).
- King David sang about the fleeting nature of life, and compared our lives to a moth and a vapor (Psalms 39:11 HCSB).
- When the Israelites returned to Israel after 70 years of captivity in Babylon, they entered a time of peace, during which they were able to rebuild a second temple.
- Isaiah wrote God would pour out His Spirit on Israel, and they would spring up like willows along the path of the water (Isaiah 44:4).
- The righteous will flourish like the palm trees (Psalm 92:12).
- Zechariah wrote about an angel of the Lord who stood among the myrtle trees, after they had walked throughout the earth and all was at peace (Zechariah 1:11).
- The crowd celebrated Jesus as the Prince of Peace when He made His final entry into Jerusalem on a donkey. They laid palm branches down on the ground for Him as he passed by, and they shouted "Hosanna," which means "save us" or Savior (John 12:13).
- Jesus said do not let your hearts become troubled or afraid; He was going to go prepare a room for us (John 14:27).

Historical application of myrtle and leafy woods

Scientists have discovered over 162 aromatic volatile compounds in the date palms. Compounds like alcohols, esters, aldehydes and ketones have been discovered in the genus *Phoenix dactylifera*[xlvii]

The fruit from these date trees has helped people and livestock to survive for thousands of years in the arid climate of the Middle East. Dates contain phytochemicals like carotenoids, polyphenols, flavonoids and amino acids, all of which have medicinal value. Their branches have long spines or thorns. Their long feathery leaves fold into a V-shape to allow them to hold moisture or water. Palms trees are either male or female, requiring each other to produce fruit. When pollen is transferred by either wind or insects from the male plant's stamen onto the female's stigma, this allows for the fertilization of the plant and for fruit to form. Some plants have both the stamen and the stigma, but the pollen is transferred in the same way.

Another occurrence in nature is when cross pollination occurs. This happens between two plants that have a different genetic structure. This can occur naturally at a very low rate, but men can also engineer plants for specific genetic traits. For example, farmers have used this process to produce hybrid grains of wheat, in order to enhance and develop being more drought tolerant.

Most of us have been taught growing up that it is better to give than to receive. This is counter intuitive unless we consider it to be like the process of pollination. When the plant releases its pollen, and in the rare exception when cross pollination occurs, the plant is transformed into something new and even possibly needed for its own and others survival. Our own Spirit is also similar to a plant because it requires an action or movement, in order to produce fruit. The Word of God cross pollinates our Spirit and transforms us in order to reproduce the fruit of eternal life.

Dates, grapes or wine, olive oil, figs, pomegranates, grains, and honey are all foods that grow in Israel. They would have been brought to the temple priests, and distributed to the orphans, widows, and sojourners during the Festival of the First Fruits. When people arrived at the temple with their part of the tithe, the priests would lead them to recite a liturgy that began with *"I have removed the sacred portion out of my house"*(Deuteronomy 26:13 ESV).

Myrtle is the type of fragrant bush that one would expect to find attracting moths at night. In the US, the Hawk Moth goes to myrtle, while in Indonesia the Rose-Myrtle-Lappet Moth is attracted to it. I could not find any documentation on a moth in the Middle East, but that doesn't mean they aren't finding myrtle there as well!

To research insects and plants worldwide, you can go to *ProjectNoah.org*.[9] This is a global citizen science self-reporting platform to where one can share, discover, and contribute by posting photographs of plants, larva, and insects that you find in your corner of the world.

In an amazing environmental connection, plants release pheromones or fragrances to attract specific insects, which will benefit the plants by pollinating them. A moth is classified as a nocturnal insect, but it is thought to be guided by light. It is drawn up by its internal navigation system using the light of the moon, and then is able to locate pheromones released by specific plants that need the moth to pollinate it. We know that the moth can also be deterred by artificial light. When this happens it may prevent the moth from locating the plant pheromones it was designed to locate; and sadly enough, it instead knocks itself out on the counterfeit light, which may even cause its death. When this happens over and over again, the plant will also suffer.

Some insects are important for the survival of plants, but others may also become their demise. Were men and women also designed to seek their Creator God in a similar way? Over and over God's word has been compared to a light. Like the moth we are being attracted by the light of the Word (the Bible), and there we can discover the fragrance of Christ. After Christ died on the cross, Paul wrote that He gave up His life like a *fragrant offering.* There are also false or lying prophets who we are told masquerade as light. They have the power to influence and deter us from receiving the genuine fragrance of our Lord, and to rise to eternal life. (2 Corinthians 11:13-14)

The Prophet Noah and the ark

---

[9] Project Noah, projectnoah.org/spottings/12813024 [Accessed 02-06-2020]

God made a covenant with Noah, by which He instructed him to build an ark (a kind of ship) to protect himself from a future catastrophe (Genesis 6:18). The world had become filled with violence so God planned a way to destroy this evil. Then He remembered Noah, who was righteous and with whom He communicated.

Noah was instructed by God to make the ark out of *gopher wood*. Although today it is an unknown name for any kind of wood, some scholars conclude that it might be cypress. Why? Because Ezekiel wrote about a ship made from cypress or juniper (Ezekiel 27:5). There are many varieties of cypress. Some varieties like Guadalupe cypress and Gowen Cypress are endangered, and many others are decreasing *(Red List)*. Cypress is rot resistant, and is so sturdy and durable that it has also been used for railroad ties, caskets, and bridges.

After Noah built the ark, God directed the animals to come into it, all at the same time. Seven pairs of clean animals and two pairs of unclean animals went into the ark, and then it rained for 40 days and nights. The ark served as a temporary home for Noah, his three sons, their four wives, and all the animals while they were in effect quarantined for one whole year. The entire time they were protected by God's covenant promise.

After they had spent a year in the ark, God instructed Noah and his family not to leave until a dove returned with an olive branch.[xlviii] The dove Noah sent out from the ark came back to him with an olive branch, and then he was able to release every creature from their quarantine. The olive branch became a symbol of hope for a future of peace for Noah and his family, and it is still used as a symbol of peace today.

A spectrum of plants once again began to replenish the earth. They filled the air with fragrant plant volatiles, which re-created an atmosphere and environment to which life could return. God put the rainbow in the sky, and used it to make another covenant promise with Noah and the creatures on the earth, that waters would never again come to destroy all of it.

> *I have set my rainbow in the clouds, and it will be a sign of the covenant between me and the earth* (Genesis 9:13 NIV).

During this time God also gave Noah permission to eat meat with the *"lifeblood"* drained out of it. He also instructed him to be accountable for the blood (or the death) of every living animal (Genesis 9:3-4). Blood was considered the essence of life for the Israelites. When an animal was put to death for consumption, it had to be done according to God's covenant law, using a process which made the meat "kosher" (Kashrut). They were to follow specific guidelines for the preparation of all foods. but particularly in the preparation of any permitted meat (Leviticus 11:3; Deuteronomy 12:21, 14:6). Cooking was a requirement for the complete removal of blood from an animal.

The connection with the death of an animal had begun in Genesis, when God took the life of an animal for its skin, and used it to clothe Adam and Eve. Now the lifeblood began to take on a deeper meaning for the spiritual clothing of mankind.

God also gave the ancient Israelites dietary laws. These laws distinguished between clean and unclean animals. Why did He do this? Perhaps to encourage self-control and improve their health. In some instances, these laws even appear to even protect the environment. For example, eating shellfish was forbidden according to the Hebraic law, and research today has revealed that oysters do an amazing job of cleaning up the waters in which they live. Where oysters have been over-harvested for food, the waters have become dangerously polluted.

The Israelite's understood that not all actions were acceptable or profitable for themselves or their community. In other Rabbinic literature the dinner table was even referred to as the temple altar. This would have been especially true for the priests, but it is true for us today as well, as we are told in the Scriptures our bodies are also the temple of God (Ephesians

2:22). What we take in also reflects the care we give to our temple body.

The coronavirus pandemic at the first of 2020 was thought to have begun after a virus mutated from caged bats for sale in an illegal "wet" market in Wuhan, China. As of this writing in the latter part of 2020, we now understand that this virus was more likely to have been spread from the Wuhan Institute of Virology. How this careless or accidental release occurred, we might never know, but as the Chinese leadership limited the Chinese people from going to other parts of China, no one restricted tens of thousands of people from flying out of China to nearly every other nation on earth where it continues to spread.

What we do know is that COVID-19 is having a devastating effect on mankind. John Hopkins Coronavirus Resource Center reported the global death toll from this has reached 108,867 with 1,777,666 cases on Easter Sunday, 2020. September 8, 2020 the universal death toll is at 974K. The total loss of life and the devastating aftermath are still yet to be determined, but in September 2020 National Public Radio (NPR.org) reported by the end of 2020 that there could be 2.8 million deaths globally. This is truly horrific.

Interestingly, bats are unclean according to Israel's dietary laws. This is not because bats are somehow "bad," but because they serve a specific role in creation that did not make them a good food choice. Descendants from Ishmael, Abraham's oldest son born from Sarah's servant Hagar, became the father of the Arab nations. They also observe these dietary restrictions, only they call their food "Halal" instead of "kosher.

Ezra and the inspiration for Sukkot

The Israelites were instructed to live by God's covenant promises, and to never forget the way of their Creator God. But the majority of the people in Israel forgot God's Law of

Love. Instead they became distracted by the worship of foreign gods and idols, which was a common practice among their neighbors. There were fights and divisions among the tribes, and the kingdom became divided against itself.

Israel also had powerful neighbors who threatened their existence: Egyptians to their south and Babylonians and Persians to their north. According to what the prophets wrote during this time, the Israelites had not lived faithfully according to God's covenant promises, so the Lord let them be overcome by their neighbors. Babylon destroyed King Solomon's great temple, along with the walls and gates around Jerusalem. Many Israelites were murdered and many others were taken as captives. During their captivity there was a remnant of people from Israel who remained faithfully patient to God and tried to live their lives accordingly.

The prophet Daniel wrote about his own captivity in Babylon when the Spirit of God gave him wisdom and an ability to predict future events. Daniel spoke about God as the *Ancient of Days* and yearned for a time when Israel could return to their homeland and resume covenant worship with the One true God, Yahweh (Daniel 7:9;13). Daniel knew that they would be homeless and have to start over again, but he and others like him never quit praying and hoping. They believed that they would eventually regain their freedom and return to Jerusalem to resume worship as a *chosen people, a royal priesthood and a holy nation*.

Over time, the Persians conquered the Babylonians, giving the Israelites yet another foreign master. Then the Lord moved the heart of the Persian King Cyrus, and Cyrus gave his blessing for some of the Israelites to be released to return to Jerusalem and begin to rebuild the temple (2 Chronicles 36). He also returned the gold and silver vessels from Solomon's temple, which the Babylonian king Nebuchadnezzar had taken when he conquered Israel. Some of the priests were also allowed to return to Israel, where they rebuilt the Altar of Burnt Offering and resumed a portion of their worship of Yahweh.

Essence of Day

After King Cyrus died, King Artaxerxes gave the great Jewish leader Nehemiah permission to return to Jerusalem to begin repair work on the walls that had surrounded Jerusalem. At that time Ezra (a Levite scribe and priest), along with Nehemiah the governor, led a spiritual revival as this group of Israelites returned to Jerusalem 70 years after their captivity (Nehemiah 8:9).

Ezra read to them from the book of Moses about the Festival of Booths, when the Israelites fled Egypt and lived-in temporary shelters in the wilderness . These shelters were made from leafy branches of myrtle, willow, and palm. As Ezra read about the history of the Passover, the people understood these Scriptures, and were moved to once again observe the Holy Day of Sukkot (or the festival of the building of the booths). They began this by gathering palms, willows, and full-leafy woods, like myrtle, for their shelters (Nehemiah 8:13-15).

The Israelite priests eventually resumed all the duties for covenant worship, as they once more began offering animal sacrifice, baking unleavened bread, making and burning the holy incense, anointing with the holy oil, and filling and lighting the lamps on a lampstand. No one knows what happened to the original gold lampstand from the tabernacle, but Jeremiah wrote about the lampstands going into Babylon (Jeremiah 52:19). If it had been returned, or another was made in its place it is likely that they would also have continued to illuminate the second temple using olive oil as a fuel.

The Ark of the Covenant was either lost or hidden by the Israelite priest's during the Babylonian capture and has never been seen again, (although some like to speculate as to where it might still be hidden). When the Most Holy Room was rebuilt, the new Ark contained the first five books of Moses (the "Torah") and the writings of the prophets. The written word would remain the single and most holy treasure reserved for the Most Holy Room in the second temple.

The Israelite Festival of Sukkot is still observed annually in Israel for seven days to commemorate these times of peace first after God miraculously led the Israelites out of Egypt, and then again when God moved King Cyrus to return the captives to Israel.

In the closing ceremonies for the Festival of Sukkot, the Israelites also finish their annual reading of the Torah. An honorary speaker, called the "Bridegroom of the law" (Torah), reads from the last few verses in Deuteronomy. When he is finished reading, another honorary speaker comes forward to read from the beginning of Genesis. This person also has the honorary title as the "Bridegroom of the Torah, and he starts reading all over again from the beginning of the Torah.[xlix]

What about the Law of God, including the Torah, today? Jesus claimed He did not come to get rid of the law but came to fulfill the law (Matthew 5:17). Here we see a beautiful image of Jesus as the Bridegroom, and the church as the bride who anticipates her groom's arrival on their wedding day. When we regard Christ as our Bridegroom, we begin to understand the relationship He desires to have with us.

> *And they reported to the Lord who was standing among the myrtle trees, "We have gone throughout the earth and found the whole world at rest and in peace."* (Zechariah 1:11 NIV).

Ezra led the Israelites into a new era of peace with their neighbors, which allowed them to re-establish covenant worship. Once again, they joyfully sang their psalms and played their harps as they returned to their work and made preparations for the coming of *"The Wonderful Counselor, Mighty God, Everlasting Father, The Prince of Peace" (Isaiah 9:6 NIV)*. Sukkot is still considered the fourth most important pilgrimage or annual holy day observed in Israel. As a beautiful reminder and tribute, it is celebrated with the construction of booths all over Israel and meeting at the foundations of what is left of Solomon's temple, only a portion of what was the temple's Western Wall.

Jesus and His preparation of a room

A few days before the crucifixion, Jesus made arrangements for the disciples to meet Him in the Upper Room for their final meal with Him. Once again, Jesus prepared the disciples for His death. How? When He established the New Covenant by breaking bread, drinking wine, and asking them to continue to do these same things in remembrance of Him. Jesus told the disciples not to worry, because He was going away to His Father's house. He told them to have faith in both His heavenly Father and in Him. Wondrously, He said He was going away to prepare a room for them, and that someday He would come back and take them with Him (John 14:2-4).

Very few of us are familiar with the traditions related to the ancient Israelite engagements and weddings. However, the disciples would have understood something more when Jesus said he was going away to "prepare a room." After a man and woman were married, in was common for the groom to take his bride to his father's household to live. The father of the groom would have arranged or chosen his son's bride, and the bride's father would have agreed on a "bride price" (Genesis 34:12). At times this could have even included oil or perfume, if the groom's family could afford It.

All the bride had to do was to accept or reject the arrangement. If she accepted, the groom's and bride's fathers would share in a glass of wine to seal the promise related to what had been agreed upon. The couple was betrothed which is considered married from this point on, even though they would not consummate the relationship until after their wedding day. When Jesus told them He would *"go prepare a room"* it would have sounded something like a pledge of marriage to the disciples.[1] Jesus even told the disciples, *"You did not choose me but I chose you"* (John 15:16).

When the time for the wedding was near and the groom's family had everything prepared for the bride, she would go through a ritual cleansing. This was an elaborate process in which she bathed in a deep stone tub, deep enough that she could totally immerse herself over her head. This could have been followed with anointing with a perfumed oil. Once she was ready, the wedding party would light oil lamps and wait for the groom's arrival. This engagement process also reminds us of John the Baptist's proclamation, when he called the people to repentance and then with baptism which John acted on with total immersion.

We do not know if the Israelite bride carried a bouquet, but it is possible. There is evidence that this was a tradition in Egypt as early as 2500 BC.[li] Bouquets full of fragrant lilies, passionflower, jasmine and gardenia may have originally been provided in Egypt for the brides to help alleviate anxiety and to stimulate her libido, as some fragrant flowers are thought to be an aphrodisiac.

When I think about the stunning white myrtle flowers beside its dark green oval leaves with its fresh, herbaceous, sweet camphor-like aroma; and the delicate flexible swinging branches of the far reaching willows, covered in slender lance shaped green hanging leaves; and the two toned silvery gray and green lance shaped leaves of the olive tree with its uniquely twisted trunk; and the palms that provide food and coverings with their fan shaped leaves, I understand that our greatest need and desire on the earth is for a safe and permanent home with perfect peace and rest. That is what Christ is preparing for each of us when we understand and say yes to our heavenly Father.

$$\approx A\Omega \approx$$

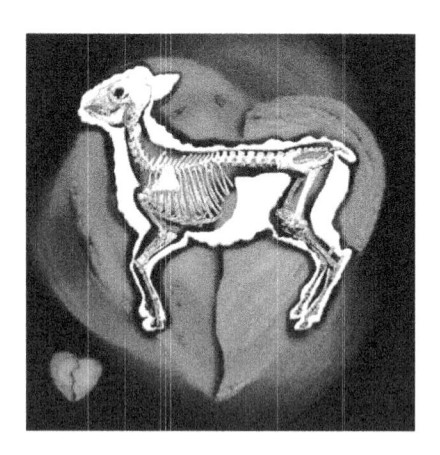

Chapter 9

Hyssop for Cleansing and Purity

Make a fragrant offering of hyssop

Hyssopus officinalis var. decumbens. This is also a common garden herb that can be potted or cut fresh.

Plant name for hyssop: *Agastache foeniculum,* or yellow hyssop, is a giant variety with a woody stem and that grows from four to seven feet tall. Giant hyssop was also harvested for its tall woody stalk.[lii]

Family: Labiatae or Lamiaceae, the same family as peppermint. With over a hundred varieties of this plant to choose from, we cannot be sure of the exact plant the Israelites used. This is mostly true for all the plants in this study. Hyssopus officinalis var. decumbens or creeping hyssop is used today for essential oils. Hyssopus officinalis is native to Southern Europe as a culinary herb. It is also used for medicinal purposes in France, Hungary and Holland, and in areas around the Caspian Sea.[liii]

Oil extraction/characteristics: EO is made by steam distillation of leaves and flower tops. It is a free-flowing pale yellow to green essential oil. Maceration of fresh cut root stems and leaves can be done in either ethanol or oil. Fresh or dried leaves can be used for cooking, or It can be boiled in water for peppermint tea.

Aroma: Hyssop has a powerful, sharp green, spicy, camphor base. A 50/50% blend of peppermint and clary sage has almost the same fragrance as hyssop if you don't have access to hyssop. Hyssop is a middle note.

Emotional benefits: Hyssop is stimulating herb. It can help to release emotional pain and grief, and may even clear mind fog.[liv]

Safety: Some types of hyssop are high in the ketones (plant chemicals) and should not be used for aromatherapy.[lv] The type of plant used in the EO should always be on the label of any purchase you make. If you ever splash an EO in your eye, remove it immediately using a small amount of oil on cotton or tissue to draw it out of the corner of your eye. Water will not work. Peppermint is in the same family as hyssop and also needs to be used with caution. Neither of these EO's are recommended for young children.

Biblical references for hyssop

- God instructed Moses to use hyssop to paint blood over the doorway of the Israelites homes at the Passover (Exodus 12:22).
- God instructed Moses about the difference between clean and unclean (Leviticus 5-7).
- Once a year, on the Day of Atonement, Moses was instructed to use hyssop, cedarwood, and scarlet wool to be burned with the red heifer. Then the ash was used to make cleansing waters (Numbers 19:6).
- Moses was instructed by God to use hyssop for sprinkling blood on the temple articles and for sprinkling or ceremonial cleansing the people of Israel (Numbers 19:18; Hebrews 9:19).
- King Solomon wrote about Hyssop (1 Kings 4:33).

- Isaiah wrote about one who was pierced for our transgressions and how He would sprinkle many nations (Isaiah 52:13-15).
- Moses used hyssop to sprinkle all the articles in the tabernacle (Hebrews 9:21).
- Jesus is the mediator of the New Covenant, whose blood was also *sprinkled* (Hebrews 12:24).

Historical application of hyssop

Hippocrates used hyssop for pleurisy and bronchitis.[lvi] It was used in the middle ages for all chest colds, lung diseases, ringing in the ears, and epilepsy.[lvii] It can be used to treat frostbite, bruises, and burns.[lviii] It is an antiseptic and a febrifuge, which means it lowers a fever. This works because of the plant alcohol content, which evaporates and thus cools the skin. It was also used to raise blood pressure, which makes it hypertensive. Hyssop is a nervine that helps tone nerves, a vulnerary that helps heal wounds, and is a cicatrisant that helps cells to regenerate (particularly on the skin). It can also be used as a diuretic.

Giant hyssop appears to have been common and affordable in the Bible lands and some type of hyssop grew voluntarily out of walls according to King Solomon (1Kings 4:33). At the top of the hyssop stalk there is an impressive bunch of tightly knit, small cup-shaped flowers. The blooms on a mature stalk can grow up to seven inches long and taper to a point like the end of a paintbrush. Their unique shape and arrangement make it possible for the blooms to hold liquid. The plant could have been used fresh or as a dried flowerhead.

Wildcrafting is a way of collecting plants from the wild to render them into essential oils. This type of essential oil is very expensive. Taking plants from their natural undisturbed environment (which of course disturbs them) is a way to find the healthiest plants that might be harvested. These would provide for their best fragrance and purest chemical composition.

So much of our environment has become polluted with chemicals and bi-products due to the introduction of synthetic compounds. Industrialization, especially in developing countries, continues to unleash a significant toxic assault against our environment. The effects of this have entered into almost every corner of our world and home. Even during King Solomon's day there were copper mines that would have polluted the land (Deuteronomy 8:9).

Sadly, we have traded the purity of our lands, seas, and air with new products from biochemical labs. For example there are over 500 toxic materials that didn't even exist a century ago. These new products allow us to prosper, survive, and make our lives easier, but their negative effects make them a double-edged sword. The condition of our earth is not where it needs to be, or where it can be. Future population growths may cause an even greater struggle to support a good quality of life on our planet. We need to have hope for change and take steps to ensure that we can leave an environmentally welcoming home for future generations.

God appeared to King Solomon after he completed the construction of the temple and said:

> *If my people, which are called by my name humble themselves, and pray and seek my face and turn from their wicked ways, then will I hear from heaven, and will forgive their sin and will heal their land* (2 Chronicles 7:14 ESV).

We, His people, are to turn from our wickedness and pray for forgiveness. There is no getting around the need for purity at every level of life, but this all begins, first and foremost, in the life of a believer. We need to look beyond ourselves and do our part to continue to support environmental laws that make sense for both our planet and its people. The corruption from politics and the motives that drive our selfish ambitions at a personal, national, and global level have deeply wounded the earth, our health, and even the quality of our lives.

Essence of Day

Millions of US dollars have gone into research in Wuhan, China laboratories for the study of viruses, such as Covid-19. It is possible this whole pandemic event was man-made because developing and selling vaccines is so lucrative for pharmaceutical companies? God instructed the Israelites that what motivated their heart and mind was just as important as the purity of their body.

Hyssop's role in purification

The use of hyssop began when God instructed Moses to make cleansing water using the ash from the sacrifice of the red heifer. The cleansing water was used to purify the Israelites when they became unclean (Numbers 8:7; 19:9-21). A person or an object could become unclean for various reasons such as coming into contact with a human corpse, bone, or even a grave. It could occur with certain skin conditions. A person could also become unclean from coming into contact with an unclean creature (Leviticus 11).

Men and women were also expected to remain pure in their marriage bed by remaining faithful to one wife or husband. The Israelites genealogy was closely tracked through the male family line because it had been well documented that the Promised One was to be born from the tribe of Judah, and more specifically from King David's branch.

Purity of heart and mind are just as important as purity of body throughout the Bible. To seek God with all your heart is to remain pure. King David questioned who could approach God if they were not pure, and God's answer is "no one" (Psalm 24:3). God asked Hosea to marry a prostitute and love her to illustrate Israel had not remained faithful to God but He loved her anyway (Hosea 3:1). The prophet Hosea also wrote that the worship of idols pollutes the heart and makes one impure (Hosea 8:5).

So what is an idol? Anything that replaces God or takes up room in our heart or mind that keeps us from serving Him. Is our desire for God or for other things? Greed for things is what is contributing to the destruction of the earth. Materialism destroys relationships with each other as well as with our heavenly Father. Ezekiel wrote that God gave the Israelites everything and tried to cleanse them, but they were still indecent and unclean because they lusted after the Assyrian's gods and men (Ezekiel 24:13). Israel failed to remain pure and wholly devoted to Yahweh, and we can and also fall into the same sorry state when we are not careful.

One time a year, on the Day of Atonement, Moses was instructed to use a stalk of hyssop (which may have included the flowering heads of the plant) to sprinkle the blood collected from the sacrificial red heifer for forgiveness of sin. No person or material item was allowed to come before God unless they went through some kind of sanctification or purification. So God provided ways for them to be purified that included sacrifice, cedarwood and hyssop. What is required of us?

> *Indeed, under the law everything is purified with blood. and without the shedding of blood there is no forgiveness of sin* (Hebrews 9:22 ESV).

Remember the first animal who was subjected to death after Eve's and Adam's sin? Blood was shed so God could clothe them with an animal skin because for the first time they realized they were naked and this made them ashamed. It was not until after the flood when there was a food shortage that God gave Noah permission to eat meat as long as the lifeblood was removed (Genesis 9:4).

With Jesus' sacrificial death on the cross, God clothed us a second time. Isaiah wrote about a bridegroom who dressed like a priest, who had clothed him with *"garments of salvation; he has covered me with the robe of His righteousness"* (Isaiah 61:10 ESV). When we believe and confess that Jesus died for our sins, He is able to purify us with the baptism of the Spirit and clothe us in His righteousness.

> *For as the earth brings forth its sprouts, and as a garden causes what is sown in it to sprout up, so the Lord God will cause righteousness and praise to sprout up before all the nations (Isaiah 61:11 ESV).*

This is not something we can do on our own (2 Corinthians 5:21). When Jesus died and then rose from the grave, He conquered death and set aside the law that condemns us. He made it possible for us to be clothed and transformed. The use of hyssop for purification demonstrated to Israel their need for a purity that they could not achieve on their own. Their obedience to His demand for purity was essential, because they understood that their sin required an intervention from God.

> *Moses then took the blood, sprinkled it on the people, and said, this is the covenant that the Lord has made with you in accordance with all these words* (Exodus 24:8 NIV).

The prophet Jeremiah wrote that God's main desire was not for the people to sacrifice and to burn blood offerings when He brought them out of Egypt. Instead, His aspiration was for the people to listen to His voice and to walk in His ways (Jeremiah 7:22-24). The prophet Hosea wrote that all God wanted was *"steadfast love not sacrifice"* (Hosea 6:6 ESV). King Solomon wrote, *"to do righteousness and justice is more acceptable to the Lord than sacrifice"* (Proverbs 21:3 ESV).

> *God made him who had no sin to be sin for us, so that in him we might become the righteousness of God* (Corinthians 5:20 NIV).

The priests were also public health inspectors, similar to that of a physician. They inspected people who had skin inflammations, and determined when white skin was leprosy or some other skin condition. When someone had a rash, a sore, or shiny spot on their flesh, they were required to see the priest. He would decide if the sore was infectious, clean, or unclean (Leviticus 13). After Jesus healed the ten lepers, He sent them on to the priests so they could be inspected. Then there would have been a purification ceremony with blood and oil, required by the law before they could rejoin the public (Leviticus 14:1-32; Luke 17:11-19).

The priests also inspected houses for different kinds of mold, which we now understand can cause brain damage and mental disorders.[lix] If a priest decided a house was unclean, the owner would need to purge it. If the mold could not be eradicated, the priest would order the family to abandon their home (Leviticus 14:39-57). Moses' law included the use of birds' blood in freshwater with cedarwood, hyssop, and scarlet yarn for sprinkling a house to purge it of mold (Leviticus 14:51). The priests also inspected fabric. If it was found to be unclean, it would be burned (Leviticus 13:51-57; Numbers 19).

God continued what He had started with Noah when Moses was instructed in the difference between clean and unclean. God wanted the Israelites to understand that some choices might lead to disease or even premature death. God wanted His people to live by a higher standard socially, emotionally, physically, and spiritually. Many of Israel's neighbors at that time in history lived life by a different set of social and legal standards. Is it safe to assume the Ten Commandments were a reaction to what was common behavior in those days.

Without the Ten Commandments, we too will fail to see our sins. But these Commandments aren't a sign of God's anger. On the contrary, the prophets Moses, Samuel, Daniel, and Nehemiah referred to God's covenant law as the "*covenant of love.*" (Deuteronomy 7:9 NIV; 1 Kings 8:23 NIV; Nehemiah 1:5 NIV; Daniel 9:4 NIV).

> *Lord the God of the heaven, the great and awesome God, who keeps his covenant of love with those who love him and keeps his commandments* (Nehemiah 1:5 NIV).

Jesus said He did not come to abolish the Law but to fulfill it (Matthew 5:17; Galatians 6:2). He was the living embodiment of the Law. Paul was a Pharisee who studied every mark and letter in the law. He was devout, but he failed to connect Jesus to what he studied, and instead of becoming a believer in Jesus he persecuted the followers of Jesus. After Jesus' death and resurrection, Paul encountered Jesus on the road to Damascus and was blinded by a great light. After this intervention from God Paul became a devout believer, but now one with a corrected and completed understanding (Acts 9:31).

Very few followers of Jesus had a comprehension of the covenant law anything like what Paul had. For example, he would have known the law that required a woman to drink the waters of bitterness if the woman's husband suspected her of adultery and became jealous (Numbers 5:24). After Paul's conversion he complemented that law when he wrote that husbands were to love their wives like Christ loved the church, and were to wash them with water through the word (Ephesians 5:26). This was radical, because women did not get the training for reading or writing of the law like men did in those days. These words derived from Paul's understanding of the law in regard to wives and their husbands. He knew that when women also became enlightened through the reading of Word, the couples' behaviors would also change for the better. Purity in a marriage relationship has always been important to God, and to anyone who wants a rich and powerful marriage.

We desperately need purity in every area of our lives- environmentally, physically, emotionally, and spiritually. We cannot compartmentalize any impure area when it comes to our relationship with God. This is not new; God knew this when He gave Moses the law and King David understood it when the Spirit anointed him and he was inspired to write and sing the prophetic Psalms. King David sang about his own personal need for purity which he knew only God could give him. Purity was so important to God that He assigned specific laws and ways to use hyssop and other fragrant plant compounds to address it. In this way the Israelites would know and remember purity has its own unique fragrance. This is also similar to the plant compounds that connect to our olfactory receptors. When our heart and mind are pure, they connect to the receptivity of our Creator God. King David knew he had failed in his attempts to remain pure and asked God to help him when he wrote:

> *Cleanse me with hyssop, and I shall be clean; wash me, and I shall be whiter than snow* (Psalm 51:7 NIV).

Moses and the raising up of hyssop for Passover

When the nation of Israel became enslaved in Egypt, they had a great struggle, both physically and spiritually, in their long and brutal bondage. Pharaoh feared the Israelites because there were so many of them and he was afraid his people would be overrun. This was because the Israelites' families produced so many healthy children. The pharaoh responded by ordering that all Hebrew baby boys be put to death at birth by their midwives. But their midwives were God-fearing and would not do this, so the mothers and midwives hid their babies.

Moses' mother had her daughter Miriam go into action to hide baby Moses in the "bulrushes," or *Cyperus papyrus*, which are long reed-like plants with a fan-shaped, grassy top that grow along the riverbanks of the Nile. Papyrus is also used to make paper, which was used for recording some of the ancient Scriptures. When an Egyptian princess came to bathe in the privacy of the papyrus reeds, she found the infant Moses tucked into a floating basket painted with tar. The basket itself may have also been woven out of papyrus reeds, which float when bundled together. The Egyptian princess had instant compassion on Moses, and took him to raise as her own son.

As an adult, Moses became painfully aware of the injustice of the Israelites' social and religious status in Egyptian society. After he witnessed a cruel Egyptian master beating a slave, Moses murdered the Egyptian and then buried him in the sand. When Moses discovered that his actions had been witnessed, he feared punishment by the Pharaoh. This caused him to flee into the desert, where he stayed until God called him back many years later to free the Israelite slaves.

Even after God brought nine plagues against Egypt for its refusal to release the Israelites, Pharaoh would still not release them. So God instructed Moses to have each Israelite household sacrifice an unblemished year-old male lamb or goat, and to use a stalk of hyssop to wipe the animal's blood over the doorway of their home. This was to ensure that the final plague of death would pass-over and spare the lives of their firstborn children and their firstborn livestock. The lamb was to be roasted over a fire, and all of it was to be eaten in haste along with bitter herbs, unleavened bread, olive oil, and wine (Exodus 12:1-43). This was called the "Passover" meal. It is still celebrated annually for seven days as the "Festival of Unleavened Bread."

Hyssop and its presence at the cross

Hyssop was also required on the Day of Atonement, when Moses was instructed to provide a sin offering by sacrificing a red heifer. Parts of the cow with its blood were to be burned outside of camp, along with red wool, cedarwood, and hyssop. Could this red wool have been taken from the lambs sacrificed every morning at the temple? We really don't know. Anything outside of the Israelite camp was considered unclean, but the zone where the red heifer, cedarwood, hyssop, and red wool were burned was considered ceremonially clean. The ash from this sacrifice was used for purification of the cleansing waters, along with other sacraments required for the purification rituals at the tabernacle (Leviticus 16:27).

The covenant law declared that there was power in the sacrificial blood to forgive sin. The sacrifice of the red heifer was to forgive both known and unknown sins. In a similar manner, Jesus was sacrificed on the cross outside the wall of Jerusalem on the Day of Atonement. This became a powerful sign to the Gentiles who were considered "unclean" because they lived outside of the walls of Jerusalem. When Christ died in the residence of the gentiles it was an act of inclusion, and meant that they too had been incorporated into God's plan of redemption under the new covenant (Hebrews 13:12).

Think back to the Day of Atonement, when the high priest wore linen and splashed the blood of the sacrificial red heifer before the temple veil, before wiping it on the horns of the altar of incense (among other places). Joseph ben Caiaphas, the high priest who led the plot to kill Jesus, would have performed all of these sacraments for the purification of his own sin and guilt annually in the temple. Did he not see his own sin in the blood? And then, with the application of the anointing oil, his own guilt? Did he forget the requirement for his own consecration with blood for his sins, even after it had been wiped on his own ear, thumb, and big toe?

The Apostle Peter wrote that those who believe Jesus is the Son of God have now become,

> *a chosen people and a royal priesthood, a holy nation, God's special possession, that you may declare the praises of him who called you out of darkness into his wonderful light* (1 Peter 2:9 NIV).

When we come to understand our sin, and acknowledge Jesus as Lord, we too become *a chosen people and a royal priesthood*. Our personal need for purity has not vanished. In fact, it has deepened, and is being transformed through the washing of the Word and within our relationship with Jesus.

God still desires for us to be pure inside and out, but this can only be accomplished when Jesus clothes us in His righteousness.

Jesus was whipped by the Roman guards, an action which would have sprayed and sprinkled His blood in every direction. It would have left him striped and pierced. Then He was nailed to a cross, upon which the Romans raised up for all to witness.

A stalk of hyssop was used twice to offer Jesus a drink while He hung on the cross. The second time a Roman guard raised up plain wine-vinegar. Jesus drank from it and declared *"It is finished,"* and He bowed His head and died (John 19:30). Jesus, the Anointed One, had completed all that He had been sent to do.

He was taken down from the cross and quickly laid to rest so that every person had time to get home before the Sabbath. Once again, the temple priests would light the holy incense and then the lamps, while each family prepared to light their oil lamps, recite the Sabbath Day blessing, and inhale the fragrant spices that would remind them of the seventh day, when all was complete and God was at rest. 700 years before His death Isaiah wrote

> *He was led like a lamb to the slaughter* (Isaiah 53:7 NIV).

After three days and nights in the tomb, Jesus, the One Consecrated from His conception by the Spirit, rose from the dead. When we confess our sins and acknowledge that Jesus died on the cross and rose from the dead like a fragrant offering, we also become a *chosen people and a royal nation*. Jesus was our sacrificial lamb.

The Israelites failed in their attempt to follow the law of Moses, just like we may also fail in our attempt to follow the whole law both inwardly and outwardly. No amount of cedarwood, hyssop, or cleansing water can purify us. Although hyssop may be good for cleansing because of its unique chemical composition of ketones, monoterpenes and alcohol, it cannot remove the impurities caused by our sin. Hyssop was just a *copy and a shadow* of what the Lord desires to complete in you.

> *Having purified your souls by your obedience to the truth for a sincere brotherly love, love one another earnestly from a pure heart (1 Peter 1:22 ESV).*

When I breathe in the powerful sharp, green, spicy, camphor-like fragrance of hyssop, I purposely remind myself of some very important applications: it was raised up by the priests to purify and sprinkle blood on the tabernacle and on the people; it was raised up again with the blood for the Passover, as part of freeing Israel from its bondage; and it was raised two more times at the cross for my sin. Purification performed by the priests was a copy and a shadow for the refining only the Anointed One can accomplish in us.

$$\approx A\Omega \approx$$

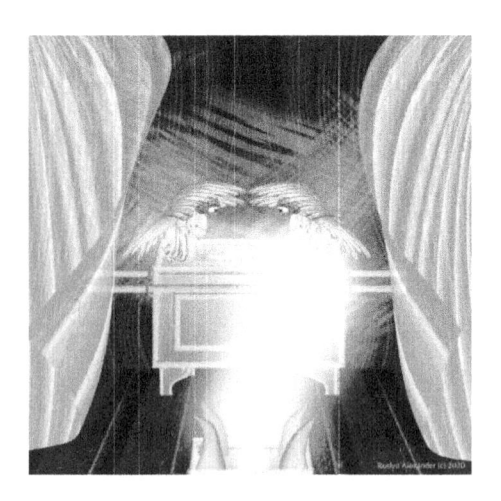

Chapter 10

Galbanum with Onycha and Our Great High Priest

Make a fragrant offering of gall and onycha

Galbanum is an herb similar to parsley and coriander. I suggest using these plants in place of fresh galbanum unless you happen to already grow this plant. Rock rose is a beautiful flower that is not familiar to most westerners. You might consider incorporating a craft project with this flower's likeness that could make a good conversation piece. This plant is prone to grow in dry sunny locations that leaves it vulnerable to fire. In the form of an EO It cost about $21.00 USD for 3 ML. I did not locate it on the Red List yet.

Plant name for gall: *Ferula galbaniflua*

Family: *Umbelliferae apiaceae.* For the purpose of this study I have chosen galbanum. It could have been the gall added to the Holy Incense. It was also a common bitter medicinal herb and was used for seasoning food. Today galbanum is processed into an exotic essential oil. Steam distillation of the plant's resin released by the stem and roots is used to make essential oil. Galbanum are from the Arabic Middle East, Iran, Turkey, Afghanistan and parts of Asia.

Plant name for onycha: *Cistus ladanifer* which goes by the common name "rockrose".

Family: *Cistaceae.* With the translation of plant names some have been led to think that onycha may be a mollusk or shellfish from the Red Sea. I question this, because shellfish were forbidden in the Israelite diet because they were defined as unclean. For this reason I fail to understand why they would burn it in the temple, which was ceremonially pure and holy. The best information I found on this was done by Dr Curtis D. Ward, whose research indicates that onycha may be from a plant commonly called rockrose [ix]. Rockrose is a small, fragrant bush found in the Mediterranean area, and has the Latin name of *Cistus ladanifer*.[lxi] This is the most believable of all my findings. The ingredients in the holy incense included frankincense, galbanum, onycha, and gum resin (possibly gum Arabic from acacia), all of which could have either been collected by hand in the hills around Jerusalem or purchased in their local markets.

Oil extraction/characteristics of gall: The plant resin from galbanum comes from the root and base stems and is gray in color. After galbanum is processed into an essential oil it is clear to yellow-green or even brownish. The resin from the root and the stems of the plant can also be macerated in oil or ethanol. The leaves can be dried and stored for a seasoning.

Oil extraction/characteristics of onycha: Rock rose leaves and stems are boiled in water, a process which releases *gum labdanum*. Essential oil is retrieved by steam distillation of stems and leaves. The gum itself would have been used for the incense.

Aroma of gall: This plant has a strong, sharp, green, weedy, or pine-like aroma with a balsamic undertone. Galbanum in the form of an essential oil is not typically purchased for its fragrance because distillation intensifies its bitter nature.

Rarely does anyone find its fragrance pleasant. Galbanum is a top note.

Aroma of onycha: or rockrose essential oil's fragrance is warm, deep, musky, and spicy fragrance. Rockrose is a base note.

Emotional benefits of gall: are calming, and can increase concentration, fortitude, and focus.[lxii]

Emotional benefits for onycha: are used for emotional trauma, or to help those who feel empty or numb.[lxiii]

Biblical references for gall and onycha

Gall is discussed a lot in the Bible:

- Moses wrote the altar of incense "*is most holy to the Lord*" (Exodus 30:10).
- Gall was an ingredient in the Holy Incense (Exodus 30:34; 2 Chronicles 13:11).
- The Holy incense was burned daily and it was also vital for the Day of Atonement (Leviticus 16:13).
- Moses recorded that any tribe or person of Israel who might turn away from serving the Lord was a root that bore gall or wormwood, which meant a poison (bitter root), and included disbelief or stubbornness of heart (Deuteronomy 29:18; 32:32).
- The use of gall had a meaning that indicated it was somehow vital for life, when it was used to describe Job's suffering (Job 16:13).
- Wickedness that is kept secret will eventually churn in one's bowels like *"the gall of asps,"* (a venomous snake) (Job 20:14 KJV).
- A few verses later a man's "gall" was ruptured by a sword, as if gall was somehow a human life (Job 20:25).
- King David wrote a psalm about gall in his food and vinegar for his thirst (Psalm 69:21).
- An author in the Psalms asks that his prayers come before God as incense which contained gall and onycha (Psalms 141:2).
- Isaiah said woe to those who confuse sweetness for bitterness and good for evil (Isaiah 5:20).
- The prophet Jeremiah wrote that they drank gall and water because they had sinned against the Lord (Jeremiah 8:14).

- The prophet Amos asked sardonically if anyone plows the sea with oxen, and then compares justice that has been turned into poison and righteousness into bitterness (Amos 6:12).
- The mention of galbanum in Matthew is thought to be some kind of plant (Matthew 2:34).
- Matthew wrote that when Jesus hung on the cross, He refused the mixture of wine with gall (and/or myrrh) (Mathew 27:34).

Historical application of bitter herbs and gall

Moses' taught that a bitter root or "gall" represented those who turned away from the faith, or who perpetuate unbelief or toxic thought (Deuteronomy 29:18). The word gall in the original Hebrew may have meant different things, such as a plant, emotional bitterness, evil, hardship, or even poison ("wormwood"). This is the hardest of all the plants to identify in Scripture because of various ways in which "gall" is used, and how it is translated into different meanings. What we do know is that the use of the word "gall" is ancient. How? Because it is referenced in the book of Job, the oldest book in the Bible. It apparently held a deeper meaning than modern translations of the word can provide. (Revelation 8:10).

In the Babylonian Talmud gall is described as one the twelve vital organs of the human body. Two other interesting vital organs included the left and right hands and the left and right feet.[lxiv] I am sure the Israelites understood one could survive without a hand or foot. So their idea of vital might have included living life to its fullest capacity, or being able to contribute as part of the whole?

There are many types bitter herbs identified in the Bible. Some were called *maror* or in the plural *merorim* [lxv] (Lamentations 3:15). These herbs may have been from the *Compositae* or *Asteraceae* family of plants which contain a white resin in their stems like that found in the sunflower, chrysanthemum, or a type of dandelion that grows wild in Israel (Exodus 12:8; Numbers 9:11). Merorim is also the root word for woman's name Miriam or Mara.

Miriam was Moses' sister, and Mara was a name Naomi took for herself after her husband and two of her sons both died within 10 years (Ruth 1:16). Since Naomi means sweetness, we also understand from this story Ruth's bitterness was equated with loss or grief. Since many cultures choose names for their baby girls that reflect a desired character, a fragrance, or a beautiful flower we need to consider that the Israelites thought the ability to grieve was also a virtue. I think most of us would agree it still is, if we give it any thought. Even the name Mary comes from this root meaning. After all, Israel believed right from their beginnings they were lamenting over the loss of the most important relationship of all, the one with their Creator God.

Wormwood is referenced six times in the ESV Bible in the books of Proverbs, Lamentations, Amos, and Revelation. It is thought to be the plant *Artemisia absinthium* and is from the Asteraceae family of plants, like the daisy, which has a bitter white resin. This is another medicinal plant found in Northern Africa and parts of Europe. It contains thujone, a plant compound which was used as a medication, but which can be toxic. Wormwood also has a very bitter taste.

Ferula galbaniflua I selected as our fragrant offering for this chapter goes by the common name galbanum. Galbanum is a plant from the same family as our modern-day *parsley* or *coriander* but it is more powerful, bitter, and green. Galbanum is not toxic. It was used for flavoring dishes, as well as for medicinal purposes. The leaves were eaten for digestive disorders, as are mint, fennel, coriander, and cilantro. The resin was also used for medicinal purposes, and could have been added to a balm or wine. The root and stems could have been steamed in water for respiratory distress, or used as a balm that could have been applied on the chest. It was most useful for wounds or inflammations on the skin. It may be hypotensive in some cases, and lower blood pressure which typically rises when someone is in pain.

Galbanum is an exotic essential oil that is still used as a medicinal plant, primarily for wounds and nervous system disorders. Some even claim that it is an aphrodisiac. [lxvi] Since gall is nontoxic, after the leaves were dried and ground it could have been what the priests used in the holy incense to help create more smoke.

I am sure the Israelites also recognized the nutritional value of eating edible flowering plants and bitter herbs that grow in the wild. Bitter herbs help with digestion, add fiber to our diet, ward off hunger, and are rich in antioxidants.

Along with nutritional benefits, if we would incorporate tasting bitter herbs like dandelions as we tell the story of the Exodus in Sunday School, we can help create a lasting memory as our students senses also become engaged in the learning process. This would allow us to give our students something remarkable to remember, just like when they learn about what the Israelites experienced in the bitterness of slavery. Not all children learn best by rote memorization, but some will thrive when given something tangible that involves their other senses.[10] Did our Creator God design sensory learning when He defined the Passover laws for Israel?

In Deuteronomy 29:18 Moses referred to a "bitter root." This had the spiritual meaning of turning away and hardening our hearts. When a bitter resin was added to any food it would embitter all of the food, making it inedible and possibly perceived as poisonous or toxic. This embitterment can also be compared to the slow toxic death of faith that can start with just one person, but can eventually infect a whole tribe or a whole nation.

Galbanum would have tasted horribly bitter and would be unpleasant to drink, but is this why Jesus refused to drink it? Seconds before Jesus' death, He was offered plain vinegar wine which He accepted (John 19:29). The ancients would have understood why this detail was significant to record,

---

[10] A note for safety: When considering plants for consumption, always refer to a reliable plant reference; ask about allergies; and get permission from parents before introducing wild or domestic plant foods; and remember that herbicides and insecticides may have been used.

Essence of Day

which leaves us asking, what was gall, and why was it important?

Recall from chapter five that Myrrh is also bitter and non-toxic. This makes it similar to galbanum as it would have also been used for medicinal purposes. *"Gall"* appears to mean to have no faith or to reject God's covenants in a way that would eventually affect everyone.

The Talmud recorded that there were many types of bitter herbs that could be used for Passover.[lxvii] What was most important was for them to taste the bitterness, rather than the type of plant that was used. So why was it important to taste the gall? For the Passover it was a way to help the Israelites to remember the bitterness of their bondage to slavery, but also the deeper bitterness of their bondage to sin and faithlessness. Other places in Scripture it was as if they were required to taste the bitterness of their sin, which was repulsive, and could cause illness or even their death.

To "have gall" appears to mean all of these qualities: to have sin and death, which results in grief, bitterness and morning. To acknowledge one's sin is to grieve over those mistakes, which should lead one to confess and repent from them. To have gall is to continue in sin due to unfaithfulness. So to remove gall would be to remove sin. Jeremiah said that those who sin, drink gall (Jeremiah 8:14)! Since we are all sinners, we all eventually drink and or serve gall in one way or another.

Jesus refused to taste the bitterness of death and stench of decay' instead, He absolutely lived-in faith and thoroughly lived His life as the Son of God. His message of eternal life is fragrant, pleasing, and sweet to our soul. He was obedient unto death in order to fulfill the law, and release us from the bitterness of slavery to sin, and eternal separation from our Creator God.

The Great High Priest and the Altar of Incense

God gave Moses directions for how to build the Altar of Incense. It was to be one-cubit square or 1.5 feet square and two cubits or 3 feet high. It was made of acacia wood with four horns on each corner and covered with gold. It also had two poles attached by rings for moving it, like the Ark of the Covenant and the Table of the Bread of Presence.

> *Once a year Aaron shall make atonement on its horns. This annual atonement must be made with the blood of the atoning sin offering for the generations to come. It is most holy unto the Lord* (Exodus 30:10 NIV).

The Altar of Incense was made from acacia wood, covered with gold and was placed just outside the Most Holy Room before the curtain or veil which shielded this most Holy part of the tabernacle. The holy incense, like the holy anointing oil, was a specific recipe that came with a harsh warning that it should not be used for any other purpose or by anyone other than the priests, or they would die (Exodus 30:33). Frankincense was the main ingredient in the holy incense that was covered in chapter two, but it is also possible dried ground galbanum leaves may have been used in the holy incense to help it create more white smoke as it burned.

If a priest or anyone in the community unintentionally sinned or did anything that was forbidden, and brought guilt to themselves, they were to sacrifice a young bull like was done for Day of Atonement, except the High priest did not enter the Most Holy Room. After the sacrifice he would sprinkle some of the blood seven times before the veil and wipe blood on the horns of the Altar of Incense (Leviticus 6:1-7). So the Altar of Incense served as a substitution for the Ark of the Covenant for the forgiveness of sin when the priest was not permitted to approach God in the Most Holy Room.

One time a year the Israelites celebrated the Day of Atonement which fell on the tenth day of the seventh month of Tishrei. The Israelite calendar used the sun and moon to calculate the twelve months for their holy days. The Roman calendar used numbers for the months and this holy day fell on the seventh month, or "September" which means seven.

The Day of Atonement is similar to the Sabbath Day, because no work was permitted, except Israel was also commanded to fast from evening to evening. The people prepared food offerings for the temple, while the high priest made preparations to meet God at the Ark of the Covenant in the Most Holy Room. The priest sacrificed a bull and sprinkled its blood before the Ark as a sin offering for himself and his household. There was also a ram (male sheep) for a burnt offering, and the people were to give two male goats to Moses. One goat was sacrificed for the sin of the people and its blood was also sprinkled, and the second goat was called the "scapegoat" and was taken to the desert and let go (Leviticus 16).

Before the priest could enter the Most Holy Room, he was required to collect live charcoal into a pan or a censor and then add two handfuls of finely ground fragrant incense to it. By adding fresh incense to the hot coals it would release the most intense fragrance while the priest entered the Most Holy Room. Wearing the required white linen and with smoke erupting from the incense, the priest approached the Ark of the Covenant. All of these steps had to be carefully completed according to the law. The fragrant veil or cloud between the priest and the Ark of the Covenant was to protect the priest so he would not die as he stood before God (Leviticus 16; Numbers 15:25; Hebrew 9:7). After all this was completed just as it is written, the people would be clean from all their sins (Leviticus 16:30).

Jesus and His role as Great High Priest

In the book of Hebrews the Altar of Incense in Herod's temple is described as being inside of the Most Holy Room. This is different from the description of where it sat in the tabernacle and King Solomon's temple. During Jesus' day we do not have an account of the exact details of how the priest entered the

Most Holy Room (Hebrews 9:4). Possibly the priest moved a part of the altar which could be separated and carried into the Most Holy Room with him? Either way, this sacrament becomes remarkable when we remember that Moses wrote that the Altar of Incense *"is most holy to the LORD"* (Exodus 30:10; Hebrews 9:7).

We are still unable to approach or see God because of our sin; however, Jesus invites each one of us to meet Him face to face. When Christ recognizes us, He makes it possible for us to approach our Creator God. Like the great high priest who was required to burn the fragrant incense to enter the Most Holy Room, we are dependent on Christ as our fragrant offering.

> *For we do not have a high priest who is unable to sympathize with our weaknesses, but one who in every respect has been tempted as we are, yet without sin* (Hebrews 4:15 ESV).

Jeremiah gave a description of a corrupted prophet's character as one who lies and is full of deceit and adultery. Many times in Scripture adultery is used to describe unfaithfulness to God. This is the same root word in our word "adulterate," which means to contaminate or ruin. This is in contrast with a true prophet, who has personal integrity, holiness and purity. A true prophet is inspired to communicate the truth directly from God to the people, even when it is not going to be popular. Jeremiah disclosed that God would require a deceitful prophet eat bitter food or drink poison (Jeremiah 23:15).

There has always been curiosity about the gall that the Roman guard offered Jesus at the cross, a drink which He refused. It is generally accepted it was a bitter plant and some think it was poison, but did it have another meaning? Perhaps it represented anything or anyone who might have been toxic or able to cause spiritual death, like the evil one. Jesus became indignant with anyone He encountered who stood in the way

Essence of Day

of God's redemption plan. For example when He rebuked Peter for suggesting that He would never be arrested, suffer and die (Matthew 16:23).

After the Passover meal, Jesus took the disciples to the Mount of Olives to pray. When they arrived, Jesus asked the disciples to stay up and pray with Him (Matthew 26:40; Mark 14:37). Besides the fact He knew He would be arrested in the early morning, there may have been another reason they were staying up all night.

On the last day of the Festival of Unleavened Bread celebrations, there may have been a tradition to stay up all night. Why? Out of gratitude for what God did for the Israelites when they were released from their bondage in Egypt. During this Feast, the story of their Exodus is retold from the beginning to the end, including the edge-of-your seat part when they were camped at the edge of the Red Sea while Pharaoh was changing his mind and sending his army out to recapture them.

Then God told Moses to raise up his staff and say,

> *Do not be afraid. Stand still, and see the salvation of the Lord, which He will accomplish for you today (Exodus 14:13 ESV).*

God parted the waters, making them into two walls, and the Israelites went through to the other side on dry ground! As the Egyptian army followed them into the seabed, the waters came back in and washed all of them away.

Only the most devoted in Israel would try and stay up all night like had happened the night God parted the waters of the Red Sea. Accumulated stress from Pharaoh's approaching army, and the East wind that blew so hard most of them would not have sleep at all in their tents anyway (Exodus 14:21).

Moses words also ring loud and clear when Jesus died on the cross. In a remarkable occurrence the temple veil shielding the Most Holy Room was torn in half. Once again God opened the way to salvation, but this time for all mankind with the blood of the true and final sacrifice of Jesus. It is interesting to note that only a priest would have been able to report this finding; since they hated Jesus, it makes the report all the more believable.

This shocking destruction of the veil would have been discovered the evening after Jesus' crucifixion. The priests' would had drawn straws to determine who would enter the Holy Room to light the Altar of Incense and then the lamps. Can you imagine his bewilderment, and then possibly his astonishment, and then perhaps at last his fear, at the realization of all that had just occurred? (Acts 6:7)

> *And walk in love, as the Messiah also loved us and gave himself for us, a sacrificial and fragrant offering to God* (Ephesians 5:2 HCSB).

Only the great high priest could receive God's forgiveness for the people's sins. The priests and religious leaders were so far from God that they actually hated Jesus for healing people and telling them, "*your sins are forgiven.*" When Jesus spoke these words, He was acting as a high priest, just as if He had carried out all the sacraments for the forgiveness of sin.

Jesus descended from the tribe of Judah, the man who was Israel's' fourth son, rather than from the tribe of Levi. What does this mean? Jesus had no birth right to claim the priesthood. But before Jacob's death, he told his sons that *"The scepter shall not depart from Judah"(Genesis 49:10).* Most priests and scribes agreed that this was a prophesy about the one who was promised to come as the Messiah. The priests had not considered that the Messiah would also serve as a high priest, even though they had been given a clue: His name meant "the Anointed One."

> *You have loved righteousness and hated wickedness; therefore God, your God, has anointed you with the oil of gladness beyond your companions* (Hebrews 1:9 ESV)

Paul explained that Jesus came from the order of Melchizedek, who was called the King of Righteousness and the King of Peace. This was the same priest whom Abraham encountered, when he offered a tithe. Strangely, Melchizedek had no earthy father or mother, and had no birthday or end of life. Instead He was like the Son of God who will serve as a priest forever (Hebrews 7:2-3 paraphrased). Some believe that Melchizedek was actually an earlier incarnation of Jesus the Christ, who wanted to walk with His people like He had with Adam and Eve.

Paul, who understood every detail of the law, wrote that Jesus is the "*exact imprint*" of God and that "*the universe is held up by His power*" (Hebrew 1:3 ESV).

Remember when the Israelites went down to Egypt in order to survive a famine, and shockingly discovered Joseph, Rachel's first-born son from Jacob (Israel)? Joseph was not only alive, but was serving as a powerful ruler, the second most powerful in all of Egypt. After testing them severely, Joseph received his brothers. He told them not to fear, because he would not use his power to punish them. He understood that his brother's actions were evil, but that God meant their bad actions for long-term good, so he could save many lives (Genesis 50:20).

When another Joseph came along many years later, a man who had been born in the tribe of Judah and descended from King David, he was betrothed to a faithful woman named Mary. When this Joseph discovered that Mary was pregnant, it was his legal right to break the betrothal, or even to have her stoned as a suspected adulteress.

Instead, an angel of the Lord came to Joseph and said, *"do not fear to take the virgin Mary as your wife for that which is conceived in her is from the Holy Spirit"* (Matthew 1:20 ESV). Mary could have appeared to be a sinner, but she was a pure vessel, one who was used in the process of God saving the lives of many.

Our difficulty in understanding this kind of ardent love does not change the fact that God loves us actively and desires a rich, deep relationship with us.

Moses knew that God had a plan to do an awesome thing for all people (Exodus 34:10). Today, we are no longer required to burn incense in order to approach God; instead, we may approach God through Christ, and our prayers, will rise like the incense with the petitions of all the faithful and patient saints (Revelation 8:4). The veil that was required in the tabernacle also reminds us that the church is the Bride of Christ. Jesus came to remove the "veil" from our eyes.

> *For to this day, at the reading of the old covenant, the same veil remains; it is not lifted because it is set aside only in Christ. But whenever a person turns to the Lord, the veil is removed* (2 Corinthians 3:14-18 HCSB).

I can only imagine the fragrance of the holy incense as it burned in the tabernacle with its piney, fruit-like fragrance of frankincense blended with the strong, sharp, green, weedy aroma of gall and the warm, deep, musky spice of rock rose. The combination of these powerful fragrant plants created so much smoke, it would have overwhelmed the priest's sense of smell and vision. Why? So he would not be able to experience all of God's glory. The priest knew he was a sinner who could not approach God without this fragrant smoke screen of protection.

I also understand I am a sinner who may not approach God without believing and confessing that Jesus gave up His life for my sin. Neither Jesus' life nor His message is gall which will lead me to a second death; rather, He is the unadulterated truth, that will lift me up to eternal life.

> *Return, faithless people," declares the Lord, "for I am your husband. I will choose you—one from a town and two from a clan—and bring you to Zion* (Jeremiah 3:14 NIV).

$$\approx A\Omega \approx$$

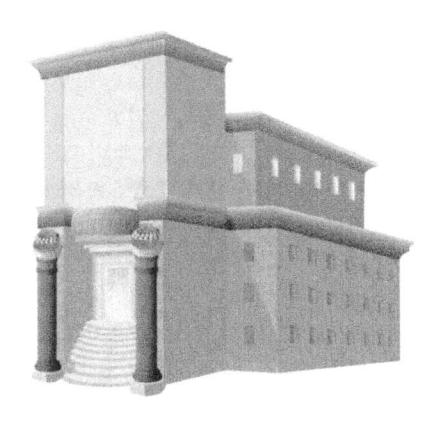

Chapter 11:

Cedarwood, Cypress, and Fir for the Temple

Make a fragrant offering of cedarwood

Substitute with *Juniperus virginiana* or cedarwood oil. Cedars of Lebanon and some other types of cyprus are found on the Red List for vulnerable (VU). *Cedrus atlantica* or cedarwood atlas is on the IUCN Red List of threatened species 2013. You could substitute with any other wood oil that is not threatened. This situation can change for better or worse, so check from time to time. There are ongoing efforts being made to protect, restore, and even begin new forests in different parts of the world.

Plant name: Juniperus virginiana, cedarwood.

Family: Cupressaceae. The Latin name Cedrus originates from the Arabic word Kedron meaning "power."[lxviii] In Greek it is pronounced Kedros. Cedarwood atlas and cedarwood virginia both have amazing aromatics and are used to make EO.

Oil extraction/characteristics: Cedar essential oil is extracted from wood chips or sawdust by steam distillation. The oil from the heartwood is more aromatic, and is yellow to amber in color.

Aroma: Cedarwood has a deep, woody, camphoraceous, cresylic or balsamic, fragrance with a sweet lift. This fragrance usually evokes a strong reaction: either one enjoys it or dislikes it. The cedars of Lebanon would have provided a powerful fragrance in King Solomon's Temple, especially in its early days when the wood was fresh. Cedarwoods are base notes.

Emotional benefits for cedar: Fortifying and strengthening, used for lethargy and poor concentration.[lxix] Cedarwood oil is sedative to the nervous system, and is helpful for chronic conditions of anxiety and nervous tension.[lxx]

Biblical references for cedarwood

- Cedarwood was often used along with hyssop for purification (Leviticus 14:4).
- Cedarwood was burned with hyssop during the sacrifice of the red heifer (Leviticus 14:52).
- *"The voice of the Lord breaks the cedars"* (Psalm 29:5 KJV).
- King Solomon's temple was constructed with cedars of Lebanon. Scripture recorded how the cedars of Lebanon were transported to build King Solomon's temple (1 Kings 5:8-10).
- King David purchased the threshing floor from Araunah the Jebusite (not an Israelite) to build Solomon's temple (2 Chronicles 3:1).
- Isaiah wrote the that the sanctuary made with fragrant woods would be a place for God's feet (Isaiah 60:13).
- Paul wrote each of us are being joined together to make a temple in the Spirit of God (Ephesians 2:22).

Historical application of cedarwood

Dioscorides and Galen referred to cedar for its use in preserving the body from putrefaction after death.[lxxi]

Cedarwoods are used to treat conditions of the scalp and hair loss, and to limit too much sebum production on the scalp. It is highly antifungal and antiseptic. It can be used to treat coughs, bronchitis, and pain from rheumatism. It can even be used as an insect repellant. It was used in mummification.[lxxii] Why? Ancient peoples may have thought this wood had the power to preserve their body and soul in death.

The cedars of Lebanon are particularly tall, and cedarwood is extremely aromatic. This tree is a protected species today because it was almost used to extinction. There are cedars from other parts of the world that may not be as impressive in stature, but which have similar aromatic properties for making EO.

Cedarwood and its use in King Solomon's Temple

Before there was a centralized government and a king in Israel, the nation was ruled by judges (Ruth 1:1). The Judges warned Israel and their leaders of their shortcomings, and reminded them that their sins would have ramifications if they continued in them. Some consider Samuel, from the tribe of Levi, to be the last Judge in Israel. He served as high priest and prophet, and mediated for justice between God and Israel (1 Samuel 1; 3:1; Acts 13:20).

Over time Israel tired of the judges, and wanted a king like the other nations around them. This was in spite of the fact that God had warned them this was not a good idea. God eventually allowed them to anoint Saul as their first king (1 Samuel 8:1-21). Samuel, the last judge, was the one who anointed King Saul. After Saul was dead, Samuel anointed King David with a horn of oil, and we are told the Spirit of the Lord came upon David powerfully (1 Samuel 16:13).

Occasionally the role of prophet and king overlapped. Samuel, the judge, and King David both predicted future events which took place in Israel that defined them as prophets. King David and the prophet Daniel wrote about the Messiah, which means the One consecrated or the One having been anointed (Daniel

9:25). Both Zadok the High Priest and Nathan the prophet anointed King David's son Solomon as king (1 Kings 1:39). Elijah the prophet anointed Hazael to be the king of Syria, and Jehu to be king of Israel, and Elisha to be his own successor as prophet (1 Kings 19:15).

About 480 years after the Israelites came out of Egypt, King David desired to build a permanent temple for the Lord. However, God did not want Israel to have a temple during David's time, because they were too busy fighting wars. Instead God gave King David directions for the first temple and announced that David's son Solomon would be the one to build it. Some of the last instructions King David gave before he died were about such things as the requirements of the priests for the purification of all the holy things in the temple, and how to place the bread on the Table of the Bread of Presence (1 Kings 7:48; 1 Chronicles 23:26)

This temple was built out of cedarwood and cypress which is a type of juniper. The temple floor was made from planks of fir. The first temple reflected all the same details, duties, and purpose of the tabernacle, only on a much grander scale.

There were ten gold lampstands, with 70 lamps to be attended twice daily (1 Kings 7). There was still only one Altar of Incense and one Table of the Bread of Presence. The Most Holy Room was 20 cubits square, and held the Ark of the Covenant with the ten commandment tablets, the most holy treasure of Israel.

1 Kings describe in detail how cedars of Lebanon were supplied for the temple. King Hiram from the city of Tyre in Lebanon, supplied Solomon with the logs which were floated down the Mediterranean Sea to Jerusalem (1 Kings 5:1-11). King Solomon in return paid King Hiram with wheat and olive oil for many years in return. God's covenant laws for the consecration of the tabernacle were also honored in the first temple. When Israel followed the everlasting covenant laws including those that required the use of fragrant offerings from the sacrificial fat, bread, incense and anointing oil, God

promised to live among them, and never to abandon His people Israel (2 Chronicles 2:3-4).

It took seven years and over ten thousand men to build the temple according to the designs God gave King David (1 Kings 6:38). If you have ever walked into a newly constructed home made from pine wood and smelled the pleasing aroma, you can only begin to understand the fragrance from the cedarwood, fir, and cypress that were used in this temple's construction. It would have been refreshing and calming for the priests as they carried out their daily duties, and reflected on God's love for Israel and what all that He had done for them.

As King Solomon contemplated the time of Israel's wandering in the desert that had become stationary under his rule, he wrote, *"Who is this that cometh out of the wilderness like pillars of smoke, perfumed with myrrh and frankincense, with all the powders of the merchant?"* (Song of Songs 3:6 KJV). Solomon appeared to be wondering who they were that God loved and was making Himself known to others by their pillars of sacrificial smoke and fragrant offerings. Even Solomon in all his wisdom could not have fully understood what an awesome thing God was going to do for all of mankind, and not just for Israel.

The amount of repetitive but meaningful work in King Solomon's temple would have greatly increased as the size of the temple and the population of the priesthood had grown. The Israelites were at their peak of prestige and power in that corner of the world when the queen of Sheba (from Africa) came to visit Solomon. She brought the king 120 talents of gold and large quantities of spices: *"there came no more such abundance of spices as these which the queen of Sheba gave to King Solomon"* (1 Kings 10:10 KJV).

There were also storerooms or side rooms built into King Solomon's temple for the storage of tithes and spices (1 Kings 6:10; 1 Chronicles 9:29; Nehemiah 12:44). Spices were valuable enough that they would have been safely guarded in the temple.

King Solomon's temple had a lily blossom flower design on the top of its columns and on the brims of the ten basins (1 Kings 7; 2 Chronicles 4:8 Ten lavers (basins). The Blue Water Lily, from Egypt named *Nymphaea caerulea,* is from the plant family *Nymphaeaceae.*[lxxiii] This lily, with its beautiful blossoms that grow out of water, have a heavenly fragrance. They were once cultivated and used to make a popular perfume in Egypt. This plant is also now endangered but scientists are doing their best to bring it back.

Does it bother you that plants from surrounding countries and cultures intermingled with the culture of Israel? It should not. From day three of creation God blessed the earth so we could all observe and understand His great capacity for love and for beauty. But some people made the mistake of choosing to worship the beauty and the fragrances of creation itself. Worship of the Creator God is what made the Israelite nation unique from all of their other neighbors.

Sadly the immense prestige of Solomon's kingdom would not last long. According to the prophets, along with Israel's influence and power also came apathy for believing God's word and keeping His covenant promises. There were fights and divisions among the Israelites that split the nation. There was worship of foreign gods that corrupted the faith, broke the commandments, and eventually discarded the worship of Yahweh. Problems erupted from King Solomon's 700 wives and the 300 concubines as some of them, like the Pharaoh's daughter, who worshiped foreign gods and they turned Solomon's heart to do the same (1 Kings 3; 11:1-6).

During Israel's history there were good kings who held up the covenant law, but also those who did not follow God's plan for Israel. The Israelite King Ahaz was so wicked that he allowed Solomon's temple to become defiled with foreign idols. But then his son Hezekiah reigned 29 years, and it was written that he did what was right before the Lord. Under Hezekiah's orders, the Levites went back into the temple after it had been neglected and polluted under King Ahaz. They carried out all of the contaminating rubbish and threw it into the brook of the Kidron (2 Chronicles 29:16). Recall that the Kidron Valley was a brook that separated the Temple Mount from Mount of Olives. This valley was strategically located to also accept excess blood from the temple sacrifices that may have been plumbed to drain into it.

King Hezekiah had the temple re-consecrated for eight days before setting out the unleavened bread on the Table of the Bread of Presence (2 Chronicles 29). This was one day longer than King Solomon had consecrated it. Sometime between 716 and 687 BC Hezekiah witnessed the destruction of the Northern kingdom of Israel by the Assyrians (he was king of the Southern kingdom of Judah) (2 Kings 18).

King Solomon's temple stood for approximately 400 years, until the southern kingdom was also destroyed. This was done by the Babylonians when Zedekiah was king of Judah. Educated and skilled craftsmen were taken captive during this time, which is now referred to as "the Exile." Then King Cyrus of Persia conquered the Babylonians while the Israelites were still held there (in the land between the Tigris and the Euphrates Rivers, which is now the country of Iraq).

During this very difficult time Israel's prophets recorded some of the most compelling prophecies in all of the Bible. Ezra recorded that the prophesies of Jeremiah would be fulfilled in order that the House of the Lord in Jerusalem could be rebuilt (Ezra 1:1). During this very stressful time in Israel's history, God spoke through the prophets with some of the most specific verses written about the coming Christ.

> *Rejoice O daughter of Zion; Shout O daughter of Jerusalem: behold, thy King cometh unto thee: he is just, and having salvation; lowly, and riding upon an ass, and upon a colt the foal of an ass (Zechariah 9:9 KJV).*

The type of "productive" stress that the prophets experienced might be compared to the aromatic herbs that increase their production of oil inside the trichome cells when they suffer under harsh environmental challenges. The prophets under duress became even more inspired by the Spirit to record future events even during those very difficult social and spiritual circumstances.

Isaiah, Micah, Ezekiel, Jeremiah, and Daniel were all inspired by the Holy Spirit during their time of captivity, so that the revelation of God's plan would be continued (Isaiah 1:1; Micah 1:1). The prophet Ezra wrote that in the first year in which King Cyrus took the throne, the Spirit of God moved him to allow Israel to begin to return to Judah and begin work on their second temple (Ezra 1:1-11). God can even move the heart of a foreign king when it is time to enlist him to further God's plans.

Herod's Temple and Ezekiel's Temple

The Prophet Ezekiel told the people to renounce their idols and God would return them to Israel and accept them as a *pleasing aroma* (Ezekiel 20:41). In 538 BC King Cyrus granted permission for the Israelites to begin reconstruction of the second temple. He even returned the temple vessels that Nebuchadnezzar had carried away (Ezra 1:1-11). The governor Zerubbabel and the priest Jeshua returned to Jerusalem and rebuilt the Altar of Burnt Offering according to the pattern God gave Moses. Then the priests were able to resume the practice of animal sacrifice day by day. Once again Israel received cedars from Lebanon with a grant Cyrus provided to build the second temple.

The prophets Zechariah and Haggai encouraged the people during this time, and the temple was finished in the sixth year of King Darius. The High Priest Jeshua, along with his governor Zerubbabel completed the construction, consecration and dedication of the second temple, which would later be called Herod's temple who extensively refurbished it during his reign.

Ezra recorded that this temple was dedicated with great joy and they offered many animals for sacrifice. Ezra did not specifically mention here if the temple was consecrated with the Holy Anointing Oil and the holy incense for seven days, but he did say that the dedication was completed by the Levite priests according to what was written in the Book of Moses (Ezra 6:16-18).

Jesus Christ is also recognized as a prophet who lived during the era of the second temple, when King Herod ruled. Like the prophets of old, He primary mediated between God and Israel to restore justice to those who were marginalized, exploited and sick. Jesus was also aware of future events, and knew He would die in Jerusalem but that His words would be everlasting (Matthew 24:35). He predicted the destruction of Jerusalem when it would be surrounded by gentile armies (Luke 21:20).

This destruction happened within 40 years (a generation) after Jesus' death, when the Roman armies under Titus surrounded and eventually destroyed Jerusalem in 70 A.D. There is a memorial arch still standing in the Forum in Rome, which depicts the Romans carrying treasures from the temple in a victory parade found on the Arch of Titus in Rome. This clearly shows the seven-branch lampstand being brought into the center of Rome.

Jesus knew He would be betrayed by one of the disciples (Matthew 26:21). He knew His disciples would go into hiding after His arrest (Matthew 26:56). When Peter told Jesus that he would never leave Him, Jesus replied that Peter would deny him three times before the rooster crowed (Matthew 26:74) which was recorded he did. When Mary poured oil on Jesus, He responded that her acts of kindness would be remembered wherever the gospel was preached (Matthew 26:13).

The New Testament Scriptures contain seventeen prophecies Jesus made, which dramatically confirms that He also had the Spiritual gift of a prophecy.

The Pharisees and Sadducees argued about the texts of the prophets and had different thoughts about eternal life; for instance, the Pharisees believed in a resurrection of our bodies but the Sadducees did not. But Jesus went beyond their dry theological arguments and challenged both groups to adopt a higher standard of love and forgiveness. Why? Because Jesus understood God's plan of salvation involved the forgiveness of sin that He would extend to each one of them with His sacrificial death on the cross.

The only time that Jesus expressed intolerance was against His own religious establishment. At one point, He made a whip and drove the money changers out of the temple because they were using it as a market to sell animals for sacrifice. When Jesus was asked by what authority He performed this dramatic act, He challenged them by stating that if the temple was destroyed, that He would raise it up in three days.

Someone in the crowd responded that it took 46 years to build the temple, so how could He possibly raise it up in three days? (John 2:13-20). Now we understand that Jesus was speaking about His own death, and that the "temple" He spoke about was his own body, raised up from the grave on the third day.

On the third day of creation, God created the plants of the earth, even before there was light from the stars or planets. We cannot live without the life-giving plants on the earth, so how will we be born anew into the Kingdom of Light without being firmly planted in Jesus?

The prophet Ezekiel recorded his vision of a third temple (Ezekiel 40). Although there is a lot of speculation about this temple, which might exist in the future, the only explanation that sounds reasonable is that there will be a future time referred to in the Scriptures as a thousand years in which Christ will reign on the earth (Revelation 20:1-25). There does not appear to be a need for a physical temple in the Kingdom of God when Jesus is with us.

> *I did not see a temple in the city, because the Lord God Almighty and the Lamb are its temple* (Revelation 21:22 NIV).

The temple of God and our bodies

One day when Jesus was leaving the temple with the disciples, He told them that not one stone of the temple would be left in place, that they would all be torn down (Matthew 24:2). Today the church understands from Jesus' teachings that the Temple of God is not a building made with wood or stone, and that the church is not reserved for a single group of people, race or tribe. The church is global, and will be united as the Bride of Christ when He returns. One day we may all be surprised at whom we find present in the Kingdom, and some whom we find missing.

The Apostle Paul wrote,

> *In him the whole building is joined together and rises to become a holy temple in the Lord. And in him you too are being built together to become a dwelling in which God lives by his Spirit* (Ephesians 2:22 NIV).

The deep, woody, cresylic fragrance of cedarwood, which resists rot and insects, reminds me that I am reserved and preserved for the Day of the Lord. Then I will be awakened and lifted up into His eternal dwelling place, much like the stimulating but relaxing fragrance of cedarwood. There I will take my place within the heavenly bodies of Christ, and live forevermore (Joel 2:31; Acts 2:17-20).

> *As a young man marries a young woman, so will your Builder marry you: as a bridegroom rejoices over his*

bride, so will your God rejoice over you (Isaiah 62:5 NIV).

≈ AΩ ≈

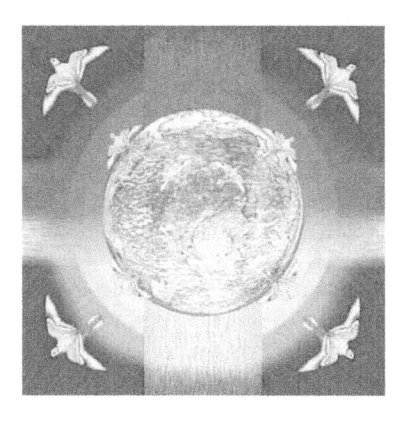

Chapter 12

Healing Leaves for the Nations

Fragrant offering of dew

Create a fragrance to be dew-like. Experiment with blends for fresh morning air, and think about why you like the fragrance. Include lemon, lime, floral, or woody fragrances, and try to find words to describe its aroma.

Aroma: There is no right or wrong fragrance for dew. The plants in your area will determine its fragrance. Consider blending top middle and base notes.

Biblical reference for leaves, healing, and sealing

- The tree of life grew in the Garden of Eden next to the tree of knowledge of good and evil.
- The Festival of Trumpets took place at the new year or Rosh Hashanah, on the first day of the seventh month (Leviticus 23:23-25).
- Ezekiel wrote about a river with water flowing from the threshold of the temple. On each side of the river grew two trees, which bear fruit every month and their leaves are for healing (Ezekiel 47:12).
- Elisha threw salt in a spring and healed the water (2 Kings 2:21).
- King Ahasuerus fixed a seal to protect the Israelites (Esther 8:8).

- David cried out to his God for help, and He healed him (Psalm 30:2).
- The valley of the shadow of death is a place we eventually all visit (Psalm 23:4).
- The lily of the valley is another plant identified in the Scriptures (Song of Solomon 2:1).
- Daniel was instructed to seal a book until the end (Daniel 12:4).
- God can heal a broken heart (Psalms 147).
- Jeremiah knew when he called on God that he would be healed and saved (Jeremiah 17:14).
- Hosea asked God's people to return to the Lord (Hosea 14:5).
- Matthew witnessed God healing many people (Matthew 4:24).
- Christ anoints us and seals us (2 Corinthians 1:21).
- When healing others Jesus would often say, *"thy sins be forgiven"* (Matthew 9:5 KJV; *Luke 5:20*).
- John wrote about seven seals that no one could open, and about two trees with leaves that will heal the nations (Revelation 5:1-9; 22:2).

Historical application of healing leaves

The gel from the Aloe vera plant has been used to treat burns, including sunburns. Dandelions have treated eczema, and have been eaten for arthritis. Catnip leaves were eaten for a toothache. Basil leaves help with flatulence. Rosemary leaves may help some with their memory. Peppermint leaves are a stimulant, and are useful for some types of headaches. Thyme, yarrow, dill, spearmint, chamomile, feverfew, and many others have all been used to help with one thing or another through the ages.

Those who study aromatherapy for wound care know there are benefits for reducing bacteria, decreasing odor, reducing inflammation and pain, increasing debridement of dead tissue, increasing formation of collagen for tissue regrowth, and reducing scarring. Many times these options are cost effective and easy to apply.

Some of these oil preparations are made from myrrh, lemon, Canadian balsam fir, lavender, melaleuca, German chamomile, niaouli, and frankincense. [lxxiv] Leaves have always been used for healing. Ezekiel and John both wrote about leaves for healing. John had a vision of two trees that grow on the sides of a river that flows from the throne of God. These trees grow fruit, and their leaves will be for the healing of the nations (Revelation 22:2; Ezekiel 47:12). All in all, leaves communicated a strong message of regeneration for the ancients, and they should for us as well.

Many different kinds of tree leaves contains hundreds of microscopic pores or valves called stomata. Each stoma along with other specialized cells help to clean our air by exchanging gases. Greenhouse gasses like carbon dioxide, water vapor, methane, and ozone are a good thing for keeping our planet warm and preventing it from freezing. However CFC's or chlorofluorocarbons which are man-made pose an even greater threat. There are mounting concerns and scientific evidence these gasses are rising to levels never reached before because of human activity and the removal of so many trees. It is difficult to measure the exact numbers of people on our planet whose lives are already being shortened from poor air quality. Nevertheless what we do know is that trees and their leaves are vital for the health of our planet as they purify our air and promote healing in many other ways as well.

The parable of the soils and the seed

The Pharisees, Sadducees, Scribes, and teachers of the law were so busy trying to interpret and enforce the law of Moses, that they misunderstood the Messiah. Sometimes the modern-day church is so busy interpreting texts, prophecies, mysteries, gender roles, knowledge, and wisdom in the Bible that we forget the application of love (1 Corinthians 13:1). These details of the law are important, but only if they are kept in perspective with God's main goals, such as the salvation of people and their resurrection from the dead.

Jesus explained in the *Parable of the Sower* that the "seed" is the Word of God. We are the soil that is either fertile or challenged. When we hear, understand and receive the word (the seed) and bury it deep within the soil of our heart, we provide it a fertile place for it take root, grow, and produce fruit (Luke 8:1-8).

The types of soil (rocky, clay or sandy) and where the seed takes root and grows will affect the life of an herb, and ultimately its aromatics. The condition of our heart is also impacted by our environment for the survival or destruction of the Word of God within us.

Extreme changes in our environment related to temperature, windstorms and rainfall, all of which vary from year to year, affects even wild or organic plants. The better the soil and the conditions, the better the chance the seed will take root and be able to survive the attacks of a fungus, virus, bacterium, insects, or a predator, so it may grow and bear fruit.

Jesus used the parable of the seed to illustrate that we can all cultivate, improve, mature, and grow, when we receive the Word of God. We do this by intentionally taking the time to listen to it, understand it, receive it, keep it safe in our hearts, and act on it when we need to remove competitors. In this way we encourage it to root, grow and bloom, so in the right season it will bear fruit. All of this planting takes faith, patience and persistence, and is never accomplished without dealing with resistance.

Resistance in the environment, on a personal level, it can come from friends, family, a local or national crisis, work, materialistic goals, or from the cultural status quo. Some nations even create laws that restrict the planting of the seed (Word), but we are still responsible to continue to cultivate the soil in our own garden (heart), regardless of the conditions, so we do not perish.

We need to acknowledge the condition of our own soil when the seed comes to us, so that change can occur. We want the coat of the seed to begin to soften, sprout, grow, bloom, and eventually bear fruit. Wherever we live on the earth, thorns, birds, rocks, and people treading on the seed are all ways Jesus used to illustrate why the seed won't take root and mature. The good soil is the person who retains the word, which exposes the darkness within themselves. Then when they confesses their sin condition, they may begin the process of cultivation so the seed will grow.

Just like in farming, the condition of our heart may change from season to season, as new environmental challenges continue to wear down our best efforts. The exception is when the Word has been allowed to become so deeply rooted in our heart and mind that we continue to act on it (the opposite is also true when sin is deeply rooted). Then, in the right season, it may sprout, grow and produce a harvest for our survival and to replenish those around us. When the word takes root and grows, it may produce a return within that individual's own lifetime, as well as for eternity.

In order for new life to spring up, the seed must first fall to the ground and die. Like Christ chose to do for us (John 12:24).

Aromatic seals and their ancient uses

A seal was a special wax used to stamp an impression of the king's signature to communicate a decree or law. Sometimes a seal was made with clay or mortar. This may have been the case with Jesus' tomb, when the Roman guards sealed it with a large rock that covered the entrance (Matthew 27:66). This could have been done by packing a mixture of mortar with clay around the seam between the stone and the tomb, and then stamping it or rolling over the whole seam with a cylinder seal to make an impression.

Other seals in Bible times were made by heating a compound of beeswax blended with fragrant tree resins that had been formed into the shape of a candle, or used as a granulated compound and heated in a metal spoon over a flame. Then it would be dripped onto paper and stamped with a custom-made metal stamp or signet ring to make an impression or insignia. The seal communicated the identity of the one who was the final authority for a decree, law or property.

Queen Esther was a woman whose Hebrew name was Hadassah, meaning myrtle. She was a beautiful young Israelite woman who had been selected by the Persian King Ahasuerus for marriage. She entered a time of preparation for her engagement with the use of cosmetic oils. This was an ancient practice, one that also commemorated the elevation of her social and legal status. [lxxv] These oils would have kept her skin soft and supple in the Mediterranean climate, and would have set her appearance apart from the common person.

When King Ahasuerus took Esther as his bride, he did not realize that she was an Israelite. How could this be? Because she had been instructed by her Uncle Mordecai to keep this a secret. Sometime after Esther's marriage there was a plot to destroy all the Jews throughout the kingdom. This plot was put together by a man named Haman, who hated them. Queen Esther found herself in a unique position to change Israel's history. At the prompting of Mordecai to act, she sought God's help by asking her people to fast and pray for three days on her behalf, after which time she would approach the king. It was against the court customs for a queen to approach a king uninvited, and he could have had her executed for this break in protocol.

After the third day, Esther approached the king, when she most certainly struggled against her own faith and fears. Happily, he welcomed her by holding out his royal scepter. Esther was then able to put into action an amazing plan God had given to her while others had prayed so she could divert the course of history for the Israelites, and it saved them. Then the king wrote an edict that protected the Jews, that could not be revoked, which he sealed with his signet ring. After all the evil Haman had planned had been exposed, the king had him executed (Esther 8:8).

The apostle John wrote that whoever believes Jesus' testimony has certified as in setting their seal, *"that God is true"* (John 3:33). John also had a vision of One seated on a throne, and in His right hand there was a scroll with seven seals. In John's vision an angel asked in a loud voice, *"'Who is worthy to open the scroll and break its seals?'"* (Revelation 5:2 ESV). Then John began to weep loudly because he knew that no one who has ever lived in all the earth was worthy to open the seals or to look at what was in the scroll. But then an elder said to John,

> *Weep no more: The Lion from the tribe of Judah, the Root of David, has conquered, so that he can open the scroll and its seven seals* (Revelation 5:5 ESV).

> *The Apostle John also wrote that when the Lamb of God opened the seventh seal, he saw seven angels who were handed seven trumpets. Then an eighth angel came and stood at an altar which is described like a heavenly altar. A golden censer was in the angel's hand and he was given an abundant amount of incense to burn in the censor, and the smoke rose with the prayers of the saints before God. After this the angel filled the censer with fire from the altar and threw it to the earth where there were shock waves from thunder, rumbling like voices and flashes of lightning* (Revelation 8:1-5 paraphrased).

Brokenness and healing

In Hebrew *Yahweh Rapha* means "the Lord That Heals." Ever since the beginning of their history, the Israelites understood that God has the power to heal.

> *But for you who revere my name, the sun of righteousness will rise with healing in its rays* (Malachi 4:2 NIV). (Exodus 15:26; 23:25).

Themes like brokenness and restoration, sickness and healing, and sin and forgiveness are present throughout the Bible. God's relationship with Adam and Eve in the Garden had been broken, but God made them clothing. The fountains of the deep were broken when Noah was in the ark, but he and his family survived. The first set of stone tablets Moses brought down from Mount Sinai were broken, but then were rewritten. Job was broken, but God restored him and his honor. When Aaron was anointed as high priest his fragrant offering of grain and oil to the Lord was to be broken (Leviticus 6:21).

Samuel the Judge wrote, *"those who oppose the Lord will be broken"* (1 Samuel 2:10 NIV). The prophet Isaiah wrote, *"the earth is defiled by its people; they disobeyed the laws, violated the statues and broke the everlasting covenant"* (Isaiah 24:5 NIV). Nevertheless Jesus came to restore us from brokenness. He broke a loaf of bread, and with it fed five thousand—and had twelve baskets of broken pieces left over! The Israelites broke God's everlasting covenant law, but Jesus came to fulfil the law and restore Himself to all peoples and nations with the new covenant.

The Pharisees accused Jesus of breaking the Sabbath when He healed a man, but Jesus taught us that the Pharisees broke justice and mercy (John 19:31). Mary broke open her alabaster perfume bottle to anoint Jesus' feet. Paul instructed the Israelites that some of them were like broken branches from an olive tree, broken off from their roots because of their unbelief, but now the gentiles had also been grafted into this tree of life (Romans 11:17-21). Only one with great authority was permitted to break open a seal and read what was written in a decree.

When you break something of great value belonging to someone else, it is reasonable and expected for you to pay them back. However, we are not able to pay back or earn back the broken relationship we have with our Creator God— only Jesus is able. Lambs sacrificed at the temple for the Passover were forbidden to have any broken bones. In a similar manner, Jesus died on the cross before the Roman guards were able to break a leg bone to speed up His death (John 19:33; 1 Samuel 2:10). What we know about our heavenly father is that,

> *He heals the brokenhearted and binds up their wounds* (Psalm 147:3 NIV).

The people in Israel witnessed Jesus restore many who had physical, emotional, and spiritual brokenness. Everywhere Jesus went He restored the sick, crippled, blind, lepers, the young, and the old. He also healed the mentally ill, social outcasts, and prostitutes. By inclusion Jesus even restored a tax collector who became the apostle Matthew.

Jesus never judged people by their sins or afflictions, instead He forgave them their sins, and taught us to do the same. He instructed the disciples to pray for the sick and anoint them with oil, which was most likely virgin olive oil. Virgin olive oil simply means the green fruit of the olive was pressed without the use of chemicals or heat. Virgin olive oil is pure, true, and unadulterated with other oils. The disciple Luke, who was also a physician, wrote at length about how Jesus healed those around Him. Luke wrote that Jesus sent out 72 disciples in pairs and instructed them to heal the sick and to say to them,

> *The kingdom of God has come near you* (Luke 10:8 ESV).

In the Old Testament three people were raised from the dead. The prophet Elijah raised the widow of Zarephath's son (1 Kings 7:17-24). Elisha raised the Shunammite's woman's son (2 Kings 4:18-37) and the Israelite man who was thrown into Elisha's tomb (2 King 13:20). In the New Testament seven people were raised from the dead, including Jesus himself.

The disciples anointed and healed many people who received a whole new understanding about the Kingdom of God and His great love for them.

Jesus rebuked illness, and healed Simon's mother-in-law (Luke 4:39). Jesus laid hands on a woman who was bent over, and she stood up (Luke 13:13). Jesus healed the blind, and said that their faith had healed them (Luke 18:43). Jesus was surprised at the faith of the Roman Centurion, who requested that Jesus even from a distance heal his servant without seeing or touching him (Luke 7:6-10). In the ultimate healing, Jesus raised His friend Lazarus from the dead (Luke 8:49-56). Ten people were raised from the dead in the Scriptures, including Jesus. The Holy Spirit continues to be active in our world today as He draws near to us for healing. This is just one of the many gifts, he bestows on His church. And yes, when we believe in Him with our whole heart, He will raise us from the dead, just as He did with Lazarus.

We are all in need of healing at one time or another emotionally, spiritually, financially, or physically. James and Mark both wrote that if anyone is sick, they should call for the elders of the church, who will pray and anoint them with oil.

> *Is anyone among you sick? Let them call the elders of the church to pray over them and anoint them with oil in the name of the Lord* (James 5:14 NIV). (Mark 16:13)

Paul taught us about the manifestations of the Holy Spirit with spiritual gifts, one of which is the gift of healing, that some receive for the common good of the church (1 Corinthians 12:9). (Psalm 103)

> *But he was pierced for our transgressions, he was crushed for our iniquities; the punishment that brought us peace was on him, and by his wounds we are healed* (Isaiah 53:5 NIV).

The ceremonial anointing with either oil or balm in the Holy Land was also used to commemorate an ascent or rise in one's legal status or with the emancipation of a slave as a relocation of property. This also included the engagement of a bride and or the legal acknowledgement of a dependent.[lxxvi]

How does that affect the way we understand the anointing of the Holy Spirit as a child of God?

> *He himself bore our sins in his body on the cross, so that we might die to sins and live for righteousness, "by his wounds you have been healed"* (1 Peter 2:24 NIV).

When Jesus returns, the earth will be liberated. Creation, along with the children of God, will be set free from the bondage of sin and death. A unique, infinite order will be established, located in a new heaven and new earth. That day will mark the first day of a new year in the Kingdom of God. Like the festival of trumpets when the Israelite's blow their shofars 100 times, this event will not go unnoticed (1 Corinthians 15:42; 51-52; 2 Peter 3:13).

> *The wolf will live with the lamb, the leopard will lie down with the goat, the calf and the lion and the yearling together; and a little child will lead them* (Isaiah 11:6 NIV).

Creation along with her children will be liberated and be restored (Romans 8:19-20). Happily on that day, plants which have been endangered will be restored, grow, bloom and bear fruit. Our physical bodies will be made new. Our hearing, sight, taste, touch and smell will be renewed to perceive in our new resurrected bodies, like we have never known before. We may even encounter a new fragrance for which we currently have no name for.

Festival of the Trumpets and the Day of the Lord

The Festival of the Trumpets takes place on the first day of the seventh month, which is also *Rosh Hashanah,* meaning the head of the new year. This holy day is commemorated by blowing horns, observing a day of rest, and making an offering of fire to the Lord. (Leviticus 23:23).

The earliest recorded event in which trumpets were sounded was at Mount Sinai after the Israelites had left Egypt. For three days, Moses consecrated the people, after they had washed their clothing. On the third day Moses went up on Mount Sinai while the Israelites stood at the base of the mountain where they heard the sound of horns blowing, and they trembled in fear. God covered the mountain in smoke and lightning and He talked to Moses in the thunder as the trumpets continued to sound. This is where God encouraged Israel to keep His covenants so that they would be a *"Kingdom of priests and a holy nation"* (Exodus 19:6 KJV).

At other places in the Scriptures shofars or animal horns made into trumpets were blown to indicate when a battle had begun. Some people think horns were also blown to announce the arrival of a groom at the home of his bride on their wedding day, but this is not verifiable in the Bible. Horns have traditionally been blown for centuries to announce one's arrival. Matthew wrote when Jesus returns it will not go unnoticed; He will send out his angels with a loud trumpet call, and they will gather His elect (Matthew 24:29).

When Jesus was asked why His disciples were eating and drinking instead of fasting and praying, Jesus answered them with a parable in which He described Himself as the bridegroom of a wedding party and when He returned, it would be as a Groom (Luke 5:34). From all over the earth those asleep in Jesus will rise out of their graves and then those living will also join Him (1 Thessalonians 4:16–17). There will be a great celebration with a banquet (Revelation 19:9).

> *The Kingdom of heaven is like a wedding banquet where a King invited many guests but only a few had even planned to attend. Then the master of the banquet sent his servants the prophets out to remind those invited to come. Instead of coming they murdered His servants. So others were invited to the banquet. They accepted the invitation gladly, put on their wedding attire and attended. One crafty guest managed to get in*

without first donning the required garment of righteousness. After he was discovered he was bound and thrown out into total darkness with the absence of all light. For many are invited but few are chosen (Matthew 22:1-14 paraphrased).

Isaiah wrote that the sorrows of this life will not be remembered in the new heaven and new earth, but instead we will rejoice for eternity (Isaiah 65:17). The apostle John was a beloved friend of Jesus who had a vision of the Kingdom of God. He saw two trees of life growing on each side of a river which flowed from the throne of God. These trees produce fruit every month of the year, and their leaves are for the healing of the nations (Revelation 22:2). What an exciting prospect that many nations will live in peace!

The healing leaves in Revelation will not just be for the personal healing of wounds, aches, pains, injuries, depression and disease. They will also be for the healing of the nations, perhaps from destruction of the environmental and economic collapse, genocides, massive social unrest, pandemics, spiritual problems, starvation, and wars, which have ruined people ever since their fall in the Garden.

The prophet Hosea pleaded with Israel to return to the Lord. He wrote that God would still love them and that His forgiveness would be like the dew in Israel, and would blossom like the lily (Hosea 14). The lily of the valley is also mentioned in the Scriptures. This might possibly be a plant similar to *Convallaria majalis*, named for its ability to thrive and grow in dappled light, wooded areas, or valleys, sometimes also called Our Lady's Tears. The plant's leaves, flowers, and berries are toxic but were at one time used as a heart medication.

It has always been one of my most favorite fragrances from nature. Its aroma is refreshing, green and lemony with a sweet, rose-like lift, an aroma I find intoxicating. This plant grows in out of the way places with its broad lush green leaves almost always covered in dew or rain drops. It has a tiny curved stem like a shepherd's staff. It shoots up with small, white, rounded, unyielding but humble, bell-shaped flowers with scalloped edging on its petals. Many of the blossoms are partially hidden within its low growing foliage. What a pleasant surprise to discover this hardy little plant's fragrance that others may have overlooked, just because of where it grows.

Like this flower, Israel itself was out of the way. Even though it was not a grand nation like its neighbors, their Holy Scriptures have changed the world.

> *I am the rose of sharon, and the lily of the valleys (Song of Solomon 2:1)*

When I take in the fragrance of the lily of the valley, I remember that one day I too will pass through the valley of the shadow of death. As I examine this great chasm that casts a shadow because of my sin, I realize my deep need for Jesus. Who humbled Himself, crossed over the Kidron Valley, bowed His head in death, but rose again to eternal life—and offers us the same.

The prophet Jeremiah grieved for his people, when he asked them why they did not turn to God for healing. He reminded them how plentiful the balm of Gilead was. *Commiphora gileadensis* is a tree that grows in Gilead, which releases a resin that was used to make a medicinal balm. It was abundant and available during that day. So Jeremiah asked why the people of Israel were not able to receive healing from God which was so very bountiful.

The people did not receive healing. Why not? Because they did not turn to God. However, God was and is still willing, ready and able to heal them (Jeremiah 8:22). Although fragrant plants and oils may be calming, healing, stimulating and enjoyable, Jehovah Rapha—"The Lord that Heals"—is the ultimate healer and lover of our souls.

> *And the leaves of the tree were for the healing of the nations. And there shall be no more curse: but the throne of God and of the Lamb shall be in it; and his servants shall serve him* (Revelation 22:2-3 NIV).

With each new day, the dew which has accumulated overnight on every herb, plant, or tree is touched by the morning light. This instantaneously heats each droplet, encouraging it to release its volatiles into the air where they are vaporized. Isaiah compared this process that the ancients understood so well, to the Day when Jesus returns and the earth gives up all of her dead.

> *But your dead will live, LORD; their bodies will rise-let those who dwell in the dust wake up and shout for joy - your dew is like the dew of the morning; the earth will give birth to her dead* (Isaiah 26:19 NIV).

When I awake in the morning and take in the sweet, fresh, herbal, green-like air, generated by the morning light which causes a release of plant volatiles, I feel rested and refreshed. The fragrances from dew remind me of the Sabbath Day of Rest, the most important holy day when happily no work was permitted. It was the Creator's passion that His One and only Son would rise for us, like a pleasing fragrance, to offer us an everlasting life, and to be ensouled in Him for all of eternity.

On the day Christ returns, I will also rise from the dead, or be caught up in the air as I am born anew into the radiant Kingdom of Light. There I am resolved to inhale the Essence of Day, when I am finally able to greet Jesus face to face.

Then Jesus will reign as Prophet, Priest, Physician, King of kings and Lord of lords forevermore.

$$\approx A\Omega \approx$$

www.facebook.com/essenceofday

Roslyn's Personal Testimony:

I was the middle child in a family of five children, and we regularly attended a Presbyterian church. When I turned 17, I decided I needed to figure out for myself what was in the Old Testament, and who Jesus was. I had heard my grandfather and father say reading the New Testament first was like putting the cart before the horse, yet in Sunday school most of my lessons had been from the New Testament.

So I began reading in Genesis, and when I got to day four, I stopped and thought, "this is either goofed up, or this is amazing. Somehow plants could grow without the energy from the sun, but instead grew with some kind of light from God?" I read it over four times and then read the rest of the Old Testament with curiosity and faith. The Word began to take root and grow and I accepted Jesus the Christ as my Lord and Savior.

In 1974, when I was a university student, I was baptized by immersion. It still surprises me that after 60+ years of life, I have never heard a pastor preach on this passage in Genesis, even though this is the passage where I tied my horse up to my spiritual cart so many years ago.

If you are interested in doing a Bible study or a workshop with these materials, or in learning more about *Essentials for Sharing the Gospel with Oil,* please contact Roslyn through her Facebook page, https://www.facebook.com/essenceofday

From 2008 to 2014, Roslyn wrote and illustrated seven children's books. Her first book, *In Seven Days?,* is about her salvation journey, a trip that ended when she became a follower of Jesus.

- All of Roslyn's children's books can be found together inside of the book *Scribe-lings,* at: https://www.lulu.com/search?adult_audience_rating=00&page=1&pageSize=10&q=Roslyn%20Alexander

- 1. *In Seven Days?* free audio book in Chinese at: youtube.com/watch?v=otWtkB4oisM.
- *In Seven Days?* (English) Published at Westbow Press. westbowpress.com/en/bookstore/bookdetails/713626-In-Seven-Days?
- 2. *Bread of Presence,* Westbow Press.
- 3. *Bones*: a free children's audio book about death, free on YouTube: youtu.be/otWtkB4oisM
- 4. *The Arks:* (Old testament for children) free audio book at: youtube.com/watch?v=Z5PMV2SxFa0
- 5. *Jonah Pursued:*
- 6. *Forty Years and Waiting:*
- 7. *Scales:*
- 8. *Blue Earth:*
-
- 10. *I Am Through the Ages:* Is an overview of the Old Testament in 30 pages, free on Smashwords: *smashwords.com/books/view/309301*

End note references

i Septimus, P., G. W., *The Project Gutenberg EBook of The Art of Perfumery. [Ebook # 16378] 2005.* http//www.gutenberg.org/files/16378/16378-h/16378-h.htm, Search: perfumery, [Accessed 01-10-2020].

ii Ecole Polytechnique Fédérale de Lausanne. *The first ever photograph of light as both a wave and a particle,* PHYS. Org, https://phys.org/news/2015-03-particle.html. 02 March 2015. [accessed 03-04-2020].

iii *Hallahan, D.L., Gray, J.C., Advances in Botanical Research Incorporation Advances in Plant Pathology, Plant Trichomes.* London, Academic Press, March 13, 2000.

iv Mojay, G., *Aromatherapy for healing the spirit.* London, Hooder and Stoughton, 1996.

v Ravindran, P.N., Divakaran, M., *Handbook of Herbs and Spices (Second Edition),* Volume 2, 2012. Science Direct, https://www.sciencedirect.com/topics/agricultural-and-biological-sciences/ruta-graveolens. [Accessed 03-2020]

vi *Red List*: https://www.iucnredlist.org/ [Accessed, 03-1-2020]

vii Mojay

viii Lawless, J., *The Encyclopedia of essential oils.* Element Books Limited, Great Britain,

ix "Ensoul." *Merriam-Webster.com Dictionary*, Merriam-Webster, https://www.merriam-webster.com/dictionary/ensoul. Accessed 11 Nov. 2020.

x 1959. Johnson, A. R., *The Vitality of the Individual in the Thought of Ancient Israel,* 1949; Buswell, J. O., *A Systematic Theology of the Christian Religion,* Zondervan, 1962, vol. 11, pp. 237-41; Wolff, H. W., *Anthropology of the Old Testament,* Sigler Pr, 1996. Seligson, M., *The Meaning of npsh* mt in the Old Testament, 1951; cf. Widengren, G., VT 4: 97-102.

xi Samuel, M. *Why did God Need to Rest on the Seventh Day?* Jewish Virtual Library, [Accessed March 16, 2020]

xii Firestein SJ, Margolskee RF, Kinnamon S. Olfaction. In: Siegel GJ, Agranoff BW, Albers RW, et al., editors. Basic Neurochemistry: Molecular, Cellular and

Medical Aspects. 6th edition. Philadelphia: Lippincott-Raven; 1999. Available from: https://www.ncbi.nlm.nih.gov/books/NBK28226/. [Accessed 08-06-2020]

xiii Rajmohan V., & Mohandas E., *The Limbic System. Indian Journal of Psychiatry,* US National Library of Medicine, National Institutes of Health, 2007 Apr-Jun; 49(2): 132–139.
Doi:10.4103/00195545.33264: https://www.ncbi.nlm.nih.gov/pmc/articles/PMC2917081/. [Accessed 03-16-2020]

xiv Battaglia, S., *The Complete Guide to Aromatherapy,* Brisbane, International Centre for Holistic Aromatherapy, 2014.

xv Cho, H. & Peterson, D.G., Ci; Exploration of Everyday Compounds, *Aroma Chemistry-The Smell of Freshly Baked Bread.*
https://www.compoundchem.com/2016/01/20/bread-aroma/. [Accessed 03-07-2020]

Cho, *Seeing the Unseen of the Combination of Two Natural Resins, Frankincense and Myrrh: Changes in Chemical Constituents and Pharmacological Activities,* NCBI. 2019 Sep; 24(17): 3076
https://www.ncbi.nlm.nih.gov/pmc/articles/PMC6749531/. [Accessed 08-05-2020]

xvi Clodovero, M.L., Camposeo, S., De Gennaro, B., Pascuzzi, S., Roselli, L., *In the Ancient World, Virgin Olive Oil was Called "Liquid Gold" by Homer and "the Great Healer" by Hippocrates. Why has this Mythic Image been Forgotten?* Science Direct, Food Research International, Volume 62, August 2014, pg. 1062-1068.
https://www.sciencedirect.com/science/article/abs/pii/S0963996914003494?via%3Dihub.%2001-23-2020. [Accessed 03-07-2020]

xvii Young, G., Encyclopedia Britannica, *Oleaceae, Plant Family,* Search: Olive tree, britannica.com/plant/Oleaceae. [Accessed 01-23-2020].

xviii Goodfellow, P. *Flora and Fauna of the Bible,* Oxford, John Beaufoy Publishing, 2015.

xix Goodfellow, P. *Flora and Fauna of the Bible,* Oxford, John Beaufoy Publishing, 2015.

xx Battaglia

xxi Williams P.A. & Phillips G.O., *Gum Arabic - an overview,* ScienceDirect, https://www.sciencedirect.com/topics/food-science/gum-arabic [accessed 03-24-2020]

xxii Arctander, S. *Perfume and flavours and material of natural origin.* Allured

xxiii Mojay

xxiv Battaglia

xxv *Grieve, M. A Modern Herbal. Penguin, UK, 1931.*

xxvi Peterfalvi, A., Miko, E., Nagy, T., Reger, B., Simon, D., Miseta, A., Czéh, B., & Szereday, L. (2019). *Much More Than a Pleasant Scent: A Review on Essential Oils Supporting the Immune System. Molecules (Basel, Switzerland)*, *24*(24), 4530. https://www.ncbi.nlm.nih.gov/pmc/articles/PMC6943609/. [Accessed 03-24-2020]

xxvii *Strong's Old Testament Hebrew Lexicon:* Search olah H5930, (KJV, public domain), https://www.biblestudytools.com/lexicons/hebrew/ [Accessed 07-15-2020]

xxviii Evans, W.C., *Trease and Evans Pharmacognosy.* 15th edn, Sydney, WD Saunders, 2002.

xxix Battaglia

xxx Caddy, R. *Essentials Oils in Colour, Caddy Classic Profiles,* Amberwood Publishing Ltd, 1997.

xxxi Mailhebiau, P. *Portraits in the Oils.* The CW. Daniel Company Limited, Great Britain, 1995.

xxxii Tisserand, R., Young, R., *Essential Oil Safety, A Guide for Health Care Professionals,* Second edition. Churchill- Livingstone-Elsevier, UK, 2002-2014.

xxxiii Battaglia

xxxiv Davis E., *Mummy Mania.* Archaeological Analysis, https://www.rsc.org/images/Archaelogical%20Analysis%20-%20Mummy%20Mania_tcm18-197541.pdf. [Accessed 03-07-2020]

xxxv Lopez-Sampson, A. & Page, T., *History of Use and Trade of Agarwood,* Springer Link, *Econ Bot* **72,** 107–129 (2018). https://doi.org/10.1007/s12231-018-9408-4, 03-20-2018. https://link.springer.com/article/10.1007/s12231-018-9408-4. [Accessed 03-07-2020]

xxxvi Battaglia

xxxvii *Gumbel, D. Principles of holistic skin therapy with herbal essences.* Karl F Haug Publishers, Germany, 1986.

xxxviii Battaglia

xxxix Lawless, J., *The Encyclopedia of essential oils.* Element Books Limited, Great Britain,

xl Worwood, V.A., *The Fragrant Heavens.* Transworld Publishing, Great Britain, 1999.

xli Buchler, A., *The Fore-Court of the Women and the Brass Gate in the Temple of Jerusalem,* JSTOR *The Jewish Quarter Review,* University of Pennsylvania Press, Vol. 10, No. 4 (Jul., 1898), pp. 678-718, https://www.jstor.org/stable/1450393?seq=1&cid=pdf-reference#references_tab_contents. [Accessed 03-07-2020]

xlii Arctander, S. *Perfume and flavours and material of natural origin.* Allured

xliii Weiss, E.A. *Essential oil Crops.* CAB International, UK, 1997.

xliv Battaglia

xlv *Gauthier, R., et al. The activity of extracts of Myrtus communis against Pediculus human capitis.* Planta Med Phytother, 1989; 23(2): 95-108. Cited in the Aromatherapy Database, Bob Harris, Essential Oil Resource Consultants, UK, 2000.

xlvi Davis, P. *Aromatherapy: An A-Z. 2nd edn.,* The C.W. Daniel Company Limited, Great Britain 1999.

xlvii *Hashim, IB; Najjar, Z; Abdulla, OA; Hassan, HM, United Arab Emirates University, UAE. Sensory flavor profiles and aromatic volatiles of six Emirati date palm fruits at three ripening stages, Argotechology,* September 11-12, 2017 San Antonio, USA. longdom.org. https://www.longdom.org/proceedings/sensory-flavor-profiles-and-aromatic-volatiles-of-six-emirati-date-palm-fruits-at-three-ripening-stages-18322.html. [Accessed 05-06-2020]

xlviii Howard, M., *How long was Noah in the Ark?* Creation Ministries International, https://creation.com/how-long-was-noah-on-the-ark. [Accessed 03-08-2020]

xlix Goodman, P., *Sukkot and Simchat Torah Anthology,* Jewish Publication Society, 1988.

l Schauss, H., *Ancient Jewish Marriage, Marriage in ancient times was a negotiated match involving an agreement on conditions and payment of a bridal price*. My Jewish Learning, https://www.myjewishlearning.com/article/ancient-jewish-marriage/ [06-14-2020].

li Belcher, B., *Creative Floral Arranging: floral designs for home and show*, Timber Press 1993. Pp 16-17. Publishing, USA, 1994.

lii Hilty, J., Yellow Giant Hyssop, Agastache nepetoides, Mint family (Lamiaceae), Illinois Wildflowers, https://www.illinoiswildflowers.info/savanna/plants/yg_hyssop.htm. [Accessed 03-09-2020]

liii Battaglia

liv Caddy, R. *Essentials Oils in Colour, Caddy Classic Profiles,* Amberwood Publishing Ltd, 1997.

lv Battaglia

lvi Le Strange, R., *A History of Herbal Plants*. Angus and Robertson, Publishers, Great Britain, 1977, 1992.

lvii *Grieve, M. A Modern Herbal. Penguin, UK, 1931*

lviii Leung, A, Foster S. *Encyclopedia of common natural ingredients used in food, drugs, and cosmetics*. 2nd end, John Wiley and Sons Inc, USA, 1996.

lix Dr. Amen, D.G., *Does Mold Affect Your Brain?* January 5, 2017, 12:57 pm, https://www.amenclinics.com/blog/toxic-mold-syndrome-it-was-like-i-lost-my-personality/ [Accessed 04-16-2020]

lx Ward, C., *What is Onycha?* Dr Curtis D. Ward, Articles and Papers, https://curtisdward.wordpress.com/2010/01/04/what-is-onycha/. [Accessed 08-05-2020].

lxi Leung, A, Foster S. *Encyclopedia of common natural ingredients used in food, drugs, and cosmetics*. 2nd end, John Wiley and Sons Inc, USA, 1996.

lxii Worwood, V.A., *The Fragrant Heavens*. Transworld Publishing, Great Britain, 1999.

lxiii Fischer-Rizzi, S., *Complete aromatherapy handbook*. Sterling Publishing Company, USA, 1990.

lxiv Davidson, W., *The William Davidson Talmud,* Sefer Yetzirah 5:2, https://www.sefaria.org/Sefer_Yetzirah.5.2?ven=Sefaria_Community_Translation&lang=bi. Search: gall [July 30:2020]

lxv *Strong's Old Testament Hebrew Lexicon:* maror 04843, (KJV, public domain), https://www.biblestudytools.com/lexicons/hebrew/ [Accessed 07-15-2020]

lxvi Leung, A, Foster S. *Encyclopedia of common natural ingredients used in food, drugs, and cosmetics.* 2nd end, John Wiley and Sons Inc, USA, 1996.

lxvii Davidson, W., *The William Davidson Talmud,* Sefer Yetzirah 5:2, https://www.sefaria.org/Sefer_Yetzirah.5.2?ven=Sefaria_Community_Translation&lang=bi. Search: gall [July 30:2020]

lxviii Mojay, G., *Aromatherapy for healing the spirit.* London, Hooder and Stoughton, 1996.

lxix Leung, A, Foster S. *Encyclopedia of common natural ingredients used in food, drugs, and cosmetics.* 2nd end, John Wiley and Sons Inc, USA, 1996.

lxx Lawless, J., *The Encyclopedia of essential oils.* Element Books Limited, Great Britain,

lxxi Ryman, D., *Aromatherapy.* Piatkus Ltd, Great Britain, 1991.

lxxii Caddy, R. *Essentials Oils in Colour, Caddy Classic Profiles,* Amberwood Publishing Ltd, 1997.

lxxiii Bertol, E., Fineschi, V., Karch, S.B., Mari, F., Riezzo, I., *Nymphaea cults in ancient Egypt and the New World: a lesson in empirical pharmacology,* Journal of the Royal Society of Medicine, J R Soc Med. 2004 Feb; 97(2): 84–85. https://www.ncbi.nlm.nih.gov/pmc/articles/PMC1079300/. [03-07-2020]

lxxiv Price, S., Price L., *Aromatherapy for Health Professionals,* Fourth edition, Churchill-Livingstone- Elsevier, UK, 1995-2014.

lxxvi Milgrom, J.; Rabinowitz, L. *"Anointing."* Encyclopaedia Judaica. Encyclopedia.com. https://www.encyclopedia.com/places/britain-ireland-france-and-low-countries/british-and-irish-political-geography/unction [Accessed 05-14-2020].

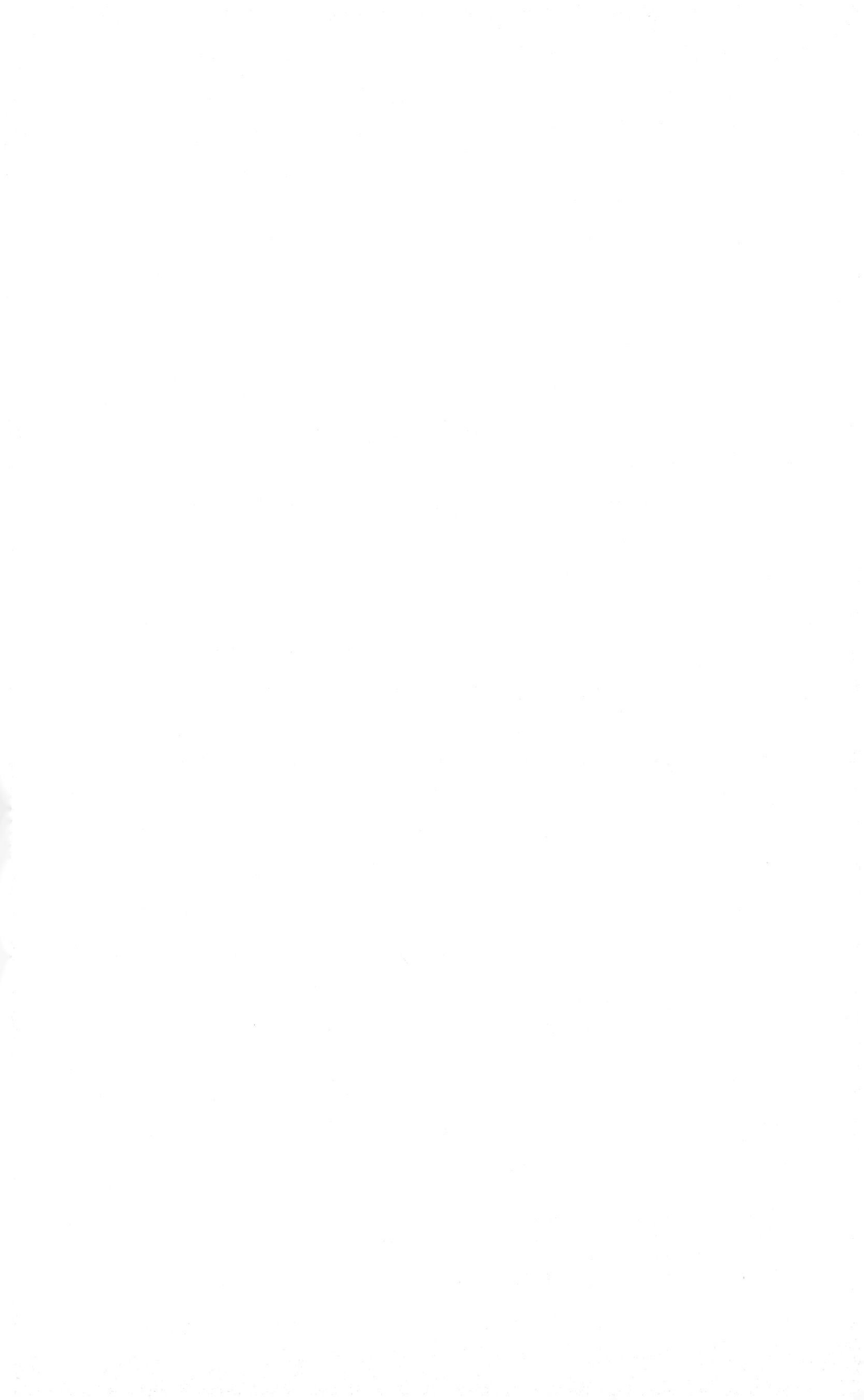

Made in the USA
Coppell, TX
03 December 2020